Legal and Ethical Issues in Health Occupations

Legal and Ethical Issues in Health Occupations

TONIA DANDRY AIKEN, R.N., B.S.N., J.D.

Attorney at Law
New Orleans, Louisiana

W.B. SAUNDERS COMPANY
A Harcourt Health Sciences Company
Philadelphia   London   New York   St. Louis   Sydney   Toronto

W.B. SAUNDERS COMPANY
A Harcourt Health Sciences Company

The Curtis Center
Independence Square West
Philadelphia, Pennsylvania 19106

Library of Congress Cataloging-in-Publication Data

Legal and ethical issues in health occupations / [edited by] Tonia D. Aiken.
 p. cm.
 ISBN 0–7216–6525–X
 1. Medical laws and legislation—United States. 2. Medical
personnel—Malpractice—United States. 3. Medical ethics. I. Aiken, Tonia D.

KF3821 .L42 2002
344.73′0412—dc21

2002049406

Publishing Director: Andrew Allen
Acquisitions Editor: Maureen Pfeifer
Developmental Editor: Rebecca Swisher
Editorial Assistant: Erin Nihill
Production Manager: Donna L. Morrissey

LEGAL AND ETHICAL ISSUES IN HEALTH OCCUPATIONS   ISBN 0–7216–6525–X

Printed in the United States of America

Last digit is the print number: 9   8   7   6   5   4   3   2   1

To my loving husband, Jim, and our wonderful children, Brett, Alexes, and Candace, who gave me support and encouragement.

To my parents, Shirley and Anthony Dandry, who taught me to reach for the sky and go after my dreams.

To Tina, Larry, Kyle, and Matthew Mayes, Julie and Courtney Bounds, Kathy Moisewicz, Jean Farquharson, Sally, Jack, Lynn and Larry Aiken, Rita, Ragus, Andrea and Ali Legendre for always being there.

And to Lavetta Ratcliff, my right hand and friend.

Contributors

James B. Aiken, M.D., M.H.A., F.A.C.E.P.,
Assistant Clinical Professor
Emergency Medicine
L.S.U. School of Medicine
President, Orleans Parish Medical
  Society;
Immediate Past-President
Louisiana Chapter
American College of Emergency
  Physicians
New Orleans, Louisiana
  *The Basics of Alternative Dispute
  Resolution*

Tonia Dandry Aiken, R.N., B.S.N., J.D.
Attorney at Law
President, Nurse Attorney Resource
  Group, Inc.
New Orleans, Louisiana
  *The Basics of Alternative Dispute
  Resolution*

Mary Powers Antoine, R.N., J.D.
Healthcare Attorney
Nossamen, Guchner, Knox & Elliot, LLP
Sacramento, California
  Informed Consent Issues

Linda Auton, R.N., J.D., R.G.
President, Advoguard Incorporated
Rockland, Massachusetts
  The Law

Nancy V. Cline, R.D.H., M.P.H.*
Dental Hygiene Education Consultant
Blanco, Texas
  *Imaging Liability and Litigation:
  Special Section on Dental Assistant
  and Hygienist*

Barbara Edwards, R.N., M.T.S.
Former Director
Cardiac Surgical Unit
Alexandria Hospital
Arlington, Virginia
  Ethical Issues in Health Occupations

Jean M. Farquharson, R.N., J.D.
Executive Director
Clinical Services and General Counsel
InterLink Home Health Services
  of Southeast Louisiana
Harvey, Louisiana
  *Intentional and Quasi-Intentional
  Torts*

Ardele Y. Float, R.N., J.D.
Attorney at Law
Law Offices of Kenneth W.
  and Ardele Y. Float
Cote de Caza, California
  Imaging Liability and Litigation

---

*Retired

vii

Kathleen M. Gialanella, R.N., J.D.
Attorney at Kathleen M.
  Gialanella, P.C.
Adjunct Professor
Seton Hall College of Nursing
South Orange, New Jersey
  *Administrative and Medical Record
  Liability and Litigation*

**Paula Dimeo Grant, R.N., B.S.N.,
M.A., J.D.**
President, Healthcare Mediators,
  Incorporated
President, Counsel, Ross & Hardies
Washington, D.C.
  *The Basics of Alternative Dispute
  Resolution*

Patricia Iyer, R.N., M.S.N.
President, Med League Support
  Services, Incorporated
Flemington, New Jersey
  *Documentation and the Allied Health
  Professional*

**Britta E. LaFont, R.D.H.,
B.A., Med.**
Assistant Professor and Clinic
  Supervisor
Program in Dental Hygiene
Department of General Dentistry
Louisiana State University School
  of Dentistry
New Orleans, Louisiana
  *Imaging Liability and Litigation:
  Special Section on Dental Assistant
  and Hygienist*

M. Lee Leppanen, R.N., J.D.
Attorney at Law
Law Offices of M. Lee Leppanen
Concord, New Hampshire
  Professional Liability Insurance

Joann Pietro, R.N., J.D.
Adjunct Associate Professor
Department of Organization
  and Leadership
Teachers College
Columbia University
New York, New York
  Patient Care Liability and Litigation

Gloria C. Ramsey, R.N., J.D.
Director
Legal and Ethical Aspects of Practice
New York University
School of Education
Division of Nursing
New York, New York
  *Legal and Ethical Issues Affecting
  Educators and Students*

Jan Simoneaux, R.N., M.N.
Campus College Chair
Department of Nursing and Health
  Sciences
University of Phoenix
Metairie, Louisiana
  *Medical Equipment Liability
  and Litigation*

**Diane Trace Warlick, R.N.,
B.S.N., J.D.**
Attorney at Law
Dallas, Texas
  *Clinical Laboratory Liability;
  The Basics of Alternative Dispute
  Resolution*

Preface

The purpose of this book is to provide allied health professionals with a textbook and reference book that focuses on the legal and ethical issues faced by them in daily practice in a user-friendly format.

The approach of this book is to provide three units that build on one another. The sections progress from basic legal principles and doctrines to specific chapters on each of the allied health professions. For example, Unit I, Legal Issues, discusses topics such as the law, intentional and quasi-intentional torts, professional liability insurance, informed consent issues, and documentation.

Unit II, Ethical Issues, is an introduction to ethical issues in health occupations and discusses those issues affecting educators and students.

Unit III, Common Areas of Liability and Litigation focuses on the individual allied health professions. For example, liability related to imaging, administrative and medical records, laboratory, medical equipment, and patient care areas are discussed. Chapter 13 is an interesting chapter entitled, "The Basics of Alternative Dispute Resolution" that focuses on the healthcare provider and the alternatives to litigation and trial.

This book is designed as a basic legal textbook for allied health professional students. The book also serves as a resource and reference book for practicing professionals in various levels and areas of health occupations.

The following are included in the chapters: key chapter concepts, objectives, introduction, case scenarios, issues, trends, ethical considerations, "boxes" of important information, pertinent points, study questions, references and resources.

This book is appropriate for: allied health professionals, students, graduate or advanced levels of allied health professionals, nurses, physicians, attorneys, administrators, and other healthcare professionals.

Tonia Dandry Aiken, R.N., B.S.N., J.D.

Acknowledgment

I want to thank the talented and knowledgeable contributors, friends and colleagues, who gave their valuable time and expertise to help in the creation of this needed text and resource book. Also, thanks to Jena Henning with the California State Department of Health Services.

Also, a warm thanks to my editors, Maureen Pfeifer, Becky Swisher, and Erin Nihill, who were instrumental in accomplishing this monumental task.

Contents

UNIT III ▶ COMMON AREAS OF LIABILITY AND LITIGATION

UNIT **I**

LEGAL ISSUES

1

The Law

LINDA AUTON, RN, JD, RG

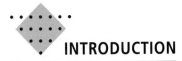

INTRODUCTION

Every job, profession, and career has a distinct vocabulary. Once familiar with the vocabulary, the ideas, concepts, and structure of the job become understandable. This chapter will review the major legal concepts and terms that will assist in understanding the rest of the concepts in the text and how those concepts affect a healthcare provider.

3

WHAT IS THE LAW?

Law is the foundation of statutes, rules, and regulations that govern people, relationships, behaviors, and interactions with the state, society, and federal government. It provides order in resolving conflicts between individuals, corporations, states, and other entities. The goal of the law is to resolve disputes without violence and protect individual citizens' health, safety, and welfare.

The law, although based on solid, long-held tenets, customs, and beliefs, is constantly evolving and growing to meet the changes, challenges, and constant shifts of our society. The past century has seen minorities become empowered by the laws changing to meet the ever-changing social, political, and personal values of society.

SOURCES OF LAW

The foundation of the law of the land is the Constitution. It grants certain powers to the federal government. If the power is not expressly granted to the federal government, then it is reserved to the state government.

The constitutional basis for federal involvement in health care is under the provision for the general welfare and regulation of interstate commerce. The states have the power to regulate health care through the state's police power to protect the health, safety, and welfare of its citizens. This includes the regulation of nurses, pharmacists, physicians, chiropractors, physical therapists, and other licensed healthcare providers.

The Constitution and the Bill of Rights guarantee certain fundamental freedoms to individuals. They impact the healthcare system by providing the fundamental rights to **privacy, equal protection, freedom of speech,** and **religion**.

The three branches of government provide the other sources of law (Box 1–1). They are the **legislative, executive,** and **judicial branches**. The first branch, the **legislature,** develops **statutory law**. These laws are codified and impact all citizens of the state. The Medicare and Medicaid amendments to the Social Security Act of 1965 have dramatically impacted health care particularly in the available services in the hospital, in the community, and at home; in hospital admissions and discharges; and in the level of care.

BOX 1-1 • FOUR SOURCES OF LAW

1. Constitution and Bill of Rights
2. Common law or case law–from the judicial branch
3. Statutory law–from the legislatures
4. Administrative law–from the executive branch

The second branch of government is the **executive branch.** The president or governor can propose laws or veto laws proposed by the legislature. They also enforce the laws and propose and establish agencies.

Agencies, under the direction of the executive branch, enact rules and regulations that become **administrative law.** Once the legislature creates a statute, it empowers the agency to implement and establish rules and regulations to meet the intent of the statute. These rules and regulations codify the interactions between the citizens and the agencies, provide for certain police power to the agencies to enforce the regulations, and govern the agencies themselves. **Occupational Safety and Health Administration (OSHA)** rules apply to most workplaces, including healthcare facilities. Another agency that regulates healthcare workplaces is the Department of Public Health (DPH), which surveys nursing homes, hospitals, and other healthcare facilities to establish regulations and enforce compliance with the regulations. The nurse practice acts of the various states create administrative agencies, such as the state boards of nursing, which have the authority to make and enforce rules and regulations concerning nursing practice.

The third branch is the **judicial system,** which develops and interprets the statutory law. It also is the source of common law, which is the law that develops from the decisions made by the court. Earlier decisions are considered **precedent** and binding on all lower courts. In Latin this is called **stare decisis,** which means to "stand by things decided" or "to adhere to decided cases."

Common law originally came from England with the Pilgrims and original settlers of the land. Since that time, each state's courts have made decisions regarding various cases, those brought by individuals in civil court as well as those brought by the state against individuals, corporations, and other entities.

CHECKS AND BALANCES

Our government has developed into three separate branches. The **executive branch** is the president of the United States or governor of an individual state. It also includes agencies that execute the laws passed by the legislature. The **legislative branch** is the **House of Representatives** and **Senate** of the United States and any similar legislature of a state. The **judicial branch** is the court system. This system includes the federal courts and the state courts.

Each branch serves as a **check and balance** for the other branches of government (Box 1–2). The legislature can develop statutes and override the veto of the president or governor. The court can declare laws developed by the legislature unconstitutional and interprets the laws. The governor or president usually can propose or veto legislation, can appoint or nominate individuals to the court, and enforces the laws. This interaction provides the checks and balances for each branch.

The legislature serves to propose and pass laws that govern the individual states, the citizens, and residents of the state and allows certain agencies to develop rules and regulations. These **rules and regulations** developed by agencies such as the Environmental Protection Agency (EPA), Board of Registration in Nursing, Board of Registration of Physicians, and OSHA apply to many employees in the health field.

The court system interprets those laws passed by the legislature as they are applied in individual cases. The court will also interpret regulations and their application to individual cases, but not until

---

BOX 1–2 • CHECKS AND BALANCES

- *Executive Branch*–president, governor–can veto legislation and enforces the laws.
- *Legislative Branch* — proposes and passes legislation; can override the president or governor.
- *Judicial Branch*–interprets legislation; can overrule laws and actions of the executive branch.

BOX 1–3 • COMMON LAW VERSUS CIVIL CODE

- *Common law*–developed on a case by case basis from England when king decided in his "divine right."
- *Civil code*–developed from Roman law codified by the legislature.

---

all remedies provided by the regulations are exhausted. For example, his employer and the Board of Registration of Pharmacists accuse Mark, who is a pharmacist, of drug diversion. After a hearing, the board suspends Mark's license as a pharmacist. Mark may appeal the case to the court. However, if there had not been a hearing, Mark could not appeal to the court, as he had not exhausted his remedies.

TYPES OF LAW

The law can be classified in many ways. One method is to look at its origins. Common law came from English common laws or written civil code (Box 1–3). These legal principles were developed when the king pronounced rules based on his "divine right." Case decisions were accumulated and based on reason and justice. All the states, but one, have adopted the common law system. Since each state adopted differing statutes and judicial interpretations, variations of the law exist between the states.

Only Louisiana, originally colonized in France, adopted a civil code based on the Napoleonic Code. The code is law created by the legislature rather than the judiciary. It is a comprehensive written set of rules and regulations rather than case by case analysis and interpretation of legal issues. It is based on Roman, Spanish, and French civil laws, not English common law.

CIVIL LAW VERSUS CRIMINAL LAW

Another way to classify law is whether there is a **civil wrong** (often called a tort) that causes harm to a person or a person's property or a **criminal wrong** that violates criminal statutes (Box 1–4).

Lawsuits against healthcare providers can be **criminal** or **civil**. The distinction is the remedy or penalty, often called a sanction.

Civil law encompasses various areas of law including but not limited to contract issues, intentional torts, negligence, malpractice, labor and privacy issues. Most cases against healthcare workers are for **negligence** or **malpractice.** The allegations in the suit are routinely that the healthcare provider failed to provide care that met the standard of care and harm resulted to the patient. The **remedies** (Box 1–5) in civil law are almost exclusively monetary. The court cannot impose servitude or make the plaintiff "whole" again when the plaintiff has suffered loss of a limb, pain, and emotional problems. The monetary award is an attempt to make the person "whole" again. On rare occasions, the court may order a person to stop doing something until a full hearing can be held on an issue. This is to prevent harm occurring that can not be remedied by money.

Criminal law is concerned with violations against society based on the criminal statutes or code. The remedies for the state or federal government are monetary fines, imprisonment and death. **Misde-meanors** are lesser crimes punishable by (usually modest) fines established by the state and/or imprisonment of less than 1 year. **Felonies** are more serious crimes punishable by much larger fines and/or imprisonment for more than 1 year and, in some states, death. In many states, a felony conviction may be the grounds for revoking a license to practice in a healthcare field. A healthcare provider may be prosecuted criminally for practicing without a license, falsifying information in obtaining a license, failing to provide life support for terminally ill patients, or patient abuse.

An agency may have both civil and criminal aspects to its rules and regulations. The remedies available encompass more than either civil

---

BOX 1–4 • CIVIL LAW VERSUS CRIMINAL LAW

- *Civil law*–case is brought by an individual or entity against another individual or entity for harm based in tort, contact, labor, or privacy issues.
- *Criminal law*–case is brought by the state or federal government for violation of written criminal code or statute.

BOX 1–5 • REMEDIES

- *Civil remedies*–usually monetary award.
- *Criminal remedies*–
  1. Misdemeanors–lesser fines and jail time of less than 1 year.
  2. Felonies–major fines and jail time of more than 1 year and the death penalty (in some states).
- *Administrative remedies*–
  1. Monetary fines
  2. Required education
  3. Loss of license to practice.

---

or criminal law. For example, the various boards of registration can suspend or revoke an individual's license to practice. It may impose educational requirements or a fine. Certain agencies may have other remedies that are specific to the agency and may vary greatly from agency to agency. For example, the Department of Public Health can suspend an institution's ability to receive Medicare or Medicaid funding, which are the major sources of funding for hospitals, rehabilitation centers, and nursing homes, as well as impose major fines. However, jail time is unusual, although Medicare and Medicaid fraud can lead to incarceration.

THE COURT SYSTEM

Each state has several levels of courts. The local courts usually deal with crimes and civil cases that do not exceed a certain minor sum established by the legislature.

The next level of court is a court with general jurisdiction. This court is the major trial court with broad powers, and it is in this court that medical malpractice, elder abuse, negligence, and other civil wrongs are tried. It is also the court where major crimes are prosecuted. Sometimes there may be specific courts set up to deal exclusively with family or probate (generally dealing with wills and administering estates when there is no will) cases, juvenile cases, housing issues, or land issues. They are limited in their jurisdiction to those cases only.

In order to try a specific case, the court must have **jurisdiction** (Box 1–6) over the case. Jurisdiction can be **in personam** or **in rem. In personam** jurisdiction means the court has jurisdiction over the person. For example, the major trial courts' jurisdiction is based on county lines or other such divisions. If the action giving rise to the case occurred in the county, the trial court in that county has jurisdiction over the case and the people involved. The plaintiff may have the option of bringing the case in his or her own county, depending on the rules of procedure for that state. In certain instances, the plaintiff may need to bring a case where the defendant lives, such as in cases involving collecting money owed.

In rem jurisdiction means the court has jurisdiction over the property or thing itself, rather than over the people involved. Right to the specific property is determined by the court and is binding usually against the whole world, not just the parties involved.

Once a trial is completed or a case is final in the court of general jurisdiction, or one of the specific courts, a case may be appealed to a higher court, usually called an **appeals court**. An **appeal** may only raise an issue of law. The facts, as found by the jury or the judge, cannot be appealed. If decided by the appeals court and no further appeal is taken, the appellate decision is binding on all lower courts in the state.

From the appeals court, an appeal may be taken to the top court of the state, usually called the **supreme court**. Again, only issues of law can be appealed. Most cases are not acted upon by the supreme court, and the parties have no recourse thereafter for further review

---

BOX 1–6 • JURISDICTION

- *In personam*–the court has jurisdiction or control over the person.
- *In rem*–the court has jurisdiction or control over the thing or property.

unless a writ of certiorari is filed with the U.S. Supreme Court and the case is chosen to be heard. The ruling by the supreme court is binding on all state courts.

Some cases may be filed in and tried by the **federal district court**. There are nine regions in the United States. The federal court hears cases that raise an issue of federal law, or the parties are from different states and the amount in controversy exceeds $75,000.00. Again, after a trial, the case may be appealed to the **federal appeals court** for that district, and then an appeal may be accepted by the **Supreme Court of the United States.**

The Justices choose cases heard by the U.S. Supreme Court. The party appealing the lower federal court's decision or a state's supreme court decision with a federal question files a petition called a "writ of certiorari." Very few cases are chosen to be heard by the U.S. Supreme Court. Those that are chosen must involve a question of substantial importance. Once the U.S. Supreme Court decides a case, it is binding on all state and federal courts.

DEFINITIONS

The case name indicates who is suing whom. The person or entity bringing the suit is called the **plaintiff**. For example, the patient who brings a complaint against the hospital, healthcare provider, or facility is the plaintiff. The person or entity who is sued is the **defendant**. An easy way to remember defendant is to think about that individual defending himself against the plaintiff's allegations. The plaintiff is listed first in the caption, such as *Jane Monroe v. ABC Hospital.*

LATIN TERMS

Certain terms in law come from Latin. The term **tort** comes from Latin, meaning to twist, be twisted, or wrest aside. It is a private or civil wrong or injury, other than breach of contract, for which the court will provide a remedy in the form of an action for damages. There must always be a violation of some duty owed to the plaintiff, and generally such duty must arise by operation of law and not by mere agreement of the parties.

Respondeat superior means "let the master answer." If a nursing assistant is sued for actions that harm a patient, her employer can also be sued. The employer can be sued on the basis that the employer had control, or should have had control, over the actions of the nursing assistant.

Res ipsa loquitur means "the thing speaks for itself." For example, a person has surgery to correct a hernia, but when he wakes up, his arm is paralyzed. Since he had no control over his actions during the surgery and a paralyzed arm is not an expected outcome or even a possible adverse reaction, then the law presumes it had to be caused by the negligence of the surgical technician, operating room nurse, surgeon or anesthesiologist. This presumption means the plaintiff does not have to prove that negligence occurred in order to recover from the defendant.

Stare decisis means literally "to stand by things decided." This prevents multiple suits on the same facts with the same parties. It allows courts to refer to previously decided similar cases and apply the same rules and principles. The courts can follow their prior decisions or those of courts of higher jurisdiction.

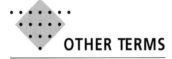

OTHER TERMS

Negligence is a tort and is a term thrown about with little thought. It is the cornerstone of a **malpractice** case. Negligence does not require a specific plan to harm someone. There are four elements in a negligence action: duty, breach, causation, and damages (Box 1–7), which will be discussed in depth later.

BOX 1–7 • ELEMENTS OF NEGLIGENCE

1. Duty
2. Breach of the duty
3. Breach the proximate/actual cause of harm
4. Harm

Malpractice requires proof of a breach of a standard of care and the breach must cause damage. Malpractice is a term used to describe the negligence of professionals, including healthcare providers. You will hear it most often in reference to nursing, medicine, and law.

Statute of limitations is used as a defense to a tort action. The statute requires that a case be brought within a specific amount of time. The requirement varies from state to state, but a suit must usually be filed within 1 to 3 years from the act or discovery of negligence or malpractice.

Insurance seems easily definable. It is a contract between the insured and the insurer that protects the insured from a specified loss. For example, a nurse anesthetist purchases a professional liability policy, also known as **malpractice insurance**, in case the nurse negligently injures a patient and is sued. The plaintiff receives only money for the injury and the insurance company pays the defense costs and any monetary award for the plaintiff. The contract merely says that in consideration for paying the policy premiums, the insurance company will make these payments on behalf of the insured.

Good Samaritan laws protect those who provide health care for an emergency or disaster without reimbursement. If a nursing assistant stops at an automobile accident and helps the victims, without seeking payment, and is not grossly negligent in rendering care, then the law covers the nursing assistant.

Sovereign immunity is a defense that protects a federal or state employee when acting within the scope of employment. The trend is to erode this defense.

Interrogatories are written questions that must be answered under oath. They are part of the discovery process, which occurs after the lawsuit is filed and before trial.

This chapter is merely a brief introduction to the terms and concepts found in this text. For further information regarding the terms, see the corresponding chapter.

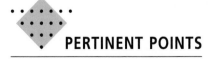

PERTINENT POINTS

1. The goal of the law is to settle disputes without violence.

2. The three branches of state and federal governments include judicial, legislative, and executive.

3. The four sources of law are the Constitution, common law, the legislature, and administrative law.

4. Plaintiff is the person or entity suing. Defendant is the person or entity sued.

5. When a plaintiff sues a defendant in a malpractice suit, it involves civil law.

6. Medical malpractice claims are based on tort theory. A tort is a civil wrong that causes harm or injury.

7. Civil law remedies provide monetary damages.

8. Criminal law remedies include fines, jail time, and possibly a death sentence.

9. Administrative law governs the rules and regulations of the different agencies and enforces them.

10. Administrative law remedies include fines, education, and loss of license to practice.

11. The legal doctrine of respondeat superior is used to pull the employer into a lawsuit because the employer is responsible and liable for the negligent acts of its employees.

12. The doctrine of res ipsa loquitur shifts the burden of proof from the plaintiffs to the defendants, who then must defend their position.

13. The good Samaritan law protects those who provide health care in an emergency without payment.

STUDY QUESTIONS

1. Discuss the reasons and goals of the law.

2. How does the law change?

3. Discuss the sources of the laws and their interactions.

4. Describe the differences between civil, criminal, and administrative law.

5. Go to the law library or use the Internet to obtain a copy of an actual case in your area of practice.

6. Describe the different levels of the judicial system.

7. Define the following terms: plaintiff, defendant, and jurisdiction. From the case you obtained, identify each.

8. What are the four elements of negligence? Underline each element you can find in the case you obtained.

9. How does the Good Samaritan law and the doctrine of sovereign immunity protect a healthcare worker?

10. Discuss the elements of a case that fall under the doctrine of res ipsa loquitur.

2

Intentional and Quasi-Intentional Torts

JEAN M. FARQUHARSON, RN, JD

▶ Objectives

At the conclusion of this chapter, the reader should have a better understanding of:

1. The nature of an intentional and quasi-intentional tort and how it differs from negligence or strict liability.

2. The necessary intent needed to commit an intentional or quasi-intentional tort.

3. The elements of assault, battery, sexual assault, false imprisonment, defamation, invasion of privacy, intentional infliction of emotional distress, and trespass to land.

4. The importance of consent and the type of consent.

5. The defenses to intentional and quasi-intentional torts.

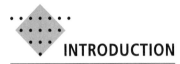

INTRODUCTION

In the day-to-day practice, healthcare professionals are confronted with situations where they must perform invasive, sometimes painful, and often humiliating procedures on their patients. Under different circumstances, these actions could give rise to legal action against the healthcare professional. While most healthcare professionals think of negligence or malpractice actions, there is another area of law where potential liability rests. It is the area known as **intentional and quasi-intentional torts.**

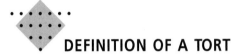

DEFINITION OF A TORT

A **tort** is a civil wrong, other than breach of contract. The word tort is derived from an old Norman word meaning "wrong." *A tort is a harm against a person, whereas a crime is a harm against the state.* For example, someone steals your purse. You make a complaint with the police, and the police arrest John Jones for the crime of theft. When that person goes to court the case is entitled *"State v. John Jones."* The state brings the action because a crime is deemed a harm against the peace and tranquillity of all persons in the state, not just against the victim.

If a tort is committed, however, it is an individual bringing the case against another individual. The state does not have an interest in seeing that you are paid money damages for any loss you sustained. In the above example, you can bring a civil action against John Jones for any loss you sustained in the theft of your purse. In such an action, you seek money damages for the loss.

Almost all torts can be crimes, but most crimes are not torts. If prison is the penalty, then the action is a crime. If money damages are the penalty, then the action is a tort.

There are four types of torts: **negligence, intentional torts, quasi-intentional torts** and **strict liability.** The essence of negligence is carelessness, whereas the essence of strict liability is the relationship to or ownership of the thing causing harm. The essence of intentional and quasi-intentional torts is consent.

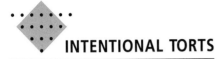

INTENTIONAL TORTS

The major intentional torts are **assault, battery, false imprisonment, intentional infliction of emotional distress,** and, in specific areas of nursing such as home care, **trespass.** Broadly defined, intentional torts require that there be an intentional interference with one's person, reputation, or property.

Intent

The degree of **intent** necessary to commit an intentional tort is broader than having a desire to bring about harm or injury to a person. If a person is or should be substantially certain that given circumstances will follow from his actions, then there is the requisite intent. For example, if you walk behind a healthcare provider in the hospital just as he pulls a tray from the dinner's cart and hits you, there is no intent to harm you, and no intentional tort is committed. But if a healthcare provider takes the tray and throws it across the room at the patient's bed, then he knew or should have known that the action of throwing a tray was likely to hit someone and cause injury. That knowledge is sufficient to form the intent necessary to commit an intentional tort.

Intent may also be transferred. For example, you intend to shoot person A, but you miss and shoot person B instead. Even though you have no intent to harm person B, your intent to harm person A is transferred, and you are deemed in law to have the intent to harm B. It is a rule of law that "intent follows the bullet." While transferred intent does not often occur in the medical setting, if a healthcare provider gives the wrong patient an injection, she can be liable for battery as well as negligence even though she has no intent to harm that patient, nor any conscious desire to administer the injection to the wrong patient.

In order to be liable for an intentional tort, a person must meet all elements of the tort. If any one element is missing, then no tort has been committed. Each of the specific torts mentioned above has specific elements, which must be met.

Assault

An **assault** means placing someone in immediate fear or apprehension of a harmful or noxious touching without the patient's consent. In order to commit an assault, the person must be aware that you are about to touch them.

For example, a patient is in bed crying and becomes hysterical. The home health aide caring for the patient becomes increasingly more anxious and upset as a result of the patient's behavior. The aide raises her hand over her head and threatens to strike the patient. (The aide does not have to tell the patient anything. Raising the hand as if to strike someone is enough.) If the patient sees the aide raising her hand and cringes to protect herself, then the patient is put in imminent fear of a battery, and the aide commits an assault.

If, on the other hand, the patient is crying into her pillow and does not see the aide raise her hand to strike, then the patient is not put in fear of an imminent battery and no assault is committed.

Usually, however, an assault precedes a battery, and the two torts are often grouped together. Keep in mind, however, that they are two separate torts.

Battery

A **battery** is defined as a harmful or offensive touching of another without his or her consent or without a legally justifiable reason. Without the consent of the patient, or absent an emergency, any touching of a patient can be a battery.

A battery does not mean you have to try and maliciously hurt or strike a person. Any touching, such as inserting an intravenous device, may be a battery if done without the consent of the person or without a legally justifiable reason. Also, hitting, spitting at, kicking, and slapping a patient can all be called batteries. In addition, you do not need to touch the patient to commit a battery. If you touch something in close proximity to the person without his or her consent, then a battery is committed. For example, if a patient wants to leave the hospital against medical advice and as the healthcare provider you grab her purse or suitcase from her hand, you have committed a battery. Even though your "intent" may have been noble, i.e., protecting her health by keeping her in the hospital, you have committed a battery.

Consent

A battery is any offensive touching without permission or in the absence of an emergency situation. All patients admitted to a hospital are required to sign a general consent. This general consent is for medical care and treatment for other employees of the hospital to "touch" the patient even in a therapeutic manner. Do not confuse this **general consent** with an **informed consent** to surgery or to other invasive procedures. While the failure to obtain an informed consent may give rise to an action in medical negligence, the consent necessary to avoid a battery is the permission to touch the person.

Battery can be committed in specific situations where there is consent to perform some procedure, but you perform another. At the cornerstone of this theory is the decision of the brilliant jurist Justice Benjamin Cardozo, who wrote in 1914,

> "Every human being of adult years and sound mind has a right to determine what shall be done with his own body, and a surgeon who performs an operation without his patient's consent commits an assault for which he is liable in damages" [1].

While you may think that no person would perform a procedure other than the one authorized, several cases are instructive. In *Pizzaloto v. Wilson* [2], the patient gave consent for the surgeon to perform exploratory surgery to accomplish lysis of adhesions and fulguration of endometriosis. During the abdominal surgery, the physician noted that Ms. Wilson's reproductive organs had sustained severe damage. He determined that she was in fact sterile and proceeded to perform a total hysterectomy and bilateral salpingo-oophrectomy.

When Ms. Wilson awoke from surgery, she was upset with what the physician had done. In ruling in her favor, the court noted, "Because no emergency was present, the surgeon committed a battery upon his patient for which Ms. Wilson is entitled to recover damages." The court awarded her $10,000. See also *Guin v. Sison* [3], where the court awarded $1000 to a postmenopausal women who had her left fallopian tube and ovary removed during the course of a colectomy. No consent was given for the salpingo-oophrectomy.

Female patients are not the only ones to be concerned. In a recent Pennsylvania case [4], plaintiff sought defendant's assistance for treatment of premature ejaculation. After conservative treatment gave only temporary relief, the defendant suggested surgery to "clear out plaque from the penis." Upon awakening from surgery, plaintiff was given a warranty card by the nurse for the penile implant the defendant had inserted during surgery. It was undisputed that no consent was given for the implant. While the trial court originally dismissed the claim because the plaintiff did not have an expert witness, the appeals court reversed and ordered the trial court to proceed with the case.

In each of the examples given, the physicians defended upon the basis that they were protecting the patients from the need for a second surgery. Even if true, and even though both surgeries were performed skillfully, the courts still held that the decision to undergo specific surgery is the plaintiffs', and absent an emergency, a physician cannot exceed the scope of the patient's consent. If the physician does so, a battery is committed.

Physicians are not the only ones who commit medical battery. Consider the facts of *Roberson v. Provident House* [5], where plaintiff, a quadriplegic, was admitted to defendant nursing home. Plaintiff wore a condom catheter, but the nursing staff obtained an order to insert a Foley catheter as needed. The order was obtained because occasionally problems developed with the condom catheter and the patient leaked urine. The physician did not discuss the insertion of a Foley catheter with the plaintiff, and the plaintiff was unaware that the order was written.

On two separate occasions the Foley catheter was inserted over the objections of the plaintiff despite his repeated requests to have the catheter removed. After the second insertion, when the plaintiff complained bitterly each shift, one nurse, who was tired of the plaintiff's complaints, jerked the catheter out, causing a discharge of blood and pus. The court found the nursing staff and their employer liable for battery. The plaintiff was awarded $25,000.

This case teaches several lessons. First and foremost, if your patient refuses to allow you to perform a procedure, STOP. If the patient objects after the fact and you can remedy the situation, then do so. In no event should any healthcare provider proceed with any procedure without the unwavering consent of the patient. Next, never perform a procedure for the convenience of the staff. That is not a reason to violate the patient's right to refuse.

Implied Consent

There are limited situations in which the courts imply consent on behalf of the plaintiff. In one of the oldest cases of implied consent, the plaintiff, an employee of defendant, spoke no English. He was standing in line with other employees to be vaccinated. He asked no questions. He watched others being vaccinated, and when it was his turn, he held up his arm to the physician who proceeded with the vaccination. When plaintiff filed suit against the company and others alleging battery, the court stated the plaintiff's action clearly implied permission to touch him. The court dismissed the battery claim [6]. It is highly unlikely that any similar situation would arise in medicine today, but there are circumstances when **consent will be implied**.

In modern medicine, consent is implied in **emergency situations**. The situation must be life threatening or pose a risk of significant physical injury to the patient if the procedures are not performed. Only those procedures absolutely necessary are authorized, and as soon as possible competent consent should be obtained. Only a physician can make the determination that a true emergency exists which necessitates proceeding without consent.

Ethical dilemmas can arise for healthcare professionals when treating individuals who, for **religious reasons**, do not allow certain procedures to be performed. If the physicians are aware of the patient's religious beliefs, then consent is not implied. If the physician is not aware, then the courts will most likely rule that the consent is implied as long as the physician had no way of knowing the religious prohibitions.

If the religious prohibitions are known, then consent is not implied, even in the case of a minor. In *Novak v. Cobb County Kennestone Hospital Authority* [7], the hospital obtained a court order to administer blood to a sixteen-year-old Jehovah's Witness. The order was entered despite the protest of the boy and his mother. Even though the mother and child brought this suit after the boy had recovered, the court dismissed all claims. Without the court order, however, the hospital and physicians could not have proceeded with the blood transfusions. Keep in mind that a court will only order the transfusions in the case of a minor. If a competent adult refuses life-saving treatment, the courts will not interfere, nor will they imply consent.

To prevent allegations of battery, always have your patient's written consent to perform a procedure. Only perform the procedure authorized, and do not exceed the scope of the consent. In emergency

situations, have at least two physicians certify that an emergency exists, document this certification in the patient's record and only perform those procedures that are necessary to save a person's life or prevent significant injury or harm. As soon as possible, obtain competent consent for the performance of additional procedures.

All states have statutes that outline when consent is implied. Healthcare providers must be aware of what their individual state laws are and, as advocates of the patient's rights, do all in their power to see to it that the law is followed.

Sexual Assault or Misconduct With Patients

The American Medical Association's Council of Ethical and Judicial Affairs has banned sexual conduct with patients under the guise of treatment in Opinion 8.14A. The American Psychiatric Association has ruled that under no circumstance is sexual activity between therapist and patient permissible. The reasons for these prohibitions are clearly illuminated in the classic case of sexual misconduct with a patient, *DiLeo v. Nugent* [8]. In *DiLeo,* plaintiff was a patient of the defendant psychiatrist for several months. In an effort to work through an impasse in therapy, the psychiatrist suggested she undergo therapy with the use of the date-rape drug, ecstasy. She and her psychiatrist had an "all day experimental session" with the plaintiff using ecstasy and tryptamine to boost the effect of ecstasy. While plaintiff was under the influence of the drug, defendant repeatedly had sexual contact with her. Defendant was found liable not only for negligence, but also willful misrepresentation. Plaintiff was awarded $500,000.

(Although plaintiff did not sue under a theory of assault and battery, the facts of DiLeo clearly support those claims.)

Psychiatrists are not the only physicians who have been sued for sexual misconduct. In *Smith v. St. Paul Fire and Marine Insurance Co.* [9], plaintiffs sued a family practitioner for sexually assaulting three boys he was treating for conditions totally unrelated to their sexual organs. In *St. Paul Fire and Marine Insurance Co. v. Asbury* [10], a gynecologist was sued by several women for fondling their clitoris during routine gynecological examinations. And in *St. Paul Fire and Marine Insurance Co. v. Shernow* [11], a dentist was sued for giving a female patient excessive doses of nitrous oxide and then sexually assaulting her. No matter what theory of liability, under no circumstances are medical practitioners, nurses or allied health personnel to have sexual relations with their patients.

False Imprisonment

False imprisonment is the unlawful detention of a person. The person is deprived of his personal liberty of movement against his will and without any authority to detain. To be falsely imprisoned, a person must be confined within a specific area against his will; he must be confined by means of physical barriers and/or by physical force or threat of physical force, and they must be aware of the confinement.

Issues of false imprisonment generally arise in three circumstances: first, in the psychiatric setting with involuntary commitments; second, with the use of restraints, either physical or chemical; and finally, in situations where a patient attempts to leave the hospital against medical advice.

In the psychiatric setting, the most important defense to a claim of false imprisonment is that all requirements in law of an involuntary admission are met. Requirements that must be met include the following:

1. The statutory provisions for the reason for involuntary commitment, such as a danger to self or others, exist

2. All statutory requirements for physician examination have been met in a timely manner.

3. All appropriate documentation exists in the chart to support the action of involuntary admit.

4. All the patient's rights have been adhered to.

5. All statutory time limits have been met but not exceeded for holding an individual against his will.

The following cases demonstrate the right and wrong ways to effect an involuntary admit.

In the case *Brand v. University Hospital* [12], the plaintiff was out of town when she became ill. She was driving to the local hospital, experienced a seizure, blacked out behind the wheel and was involved in an accident. She was transported from the scene of the accident to the local hospital. In the emergency department, the treating physician gave her the option of being admitted to neurologic service for a workup or being discharged to home to follow up with her own neurologist. Plaintiff opted for the latter.

Because of her medical condition she called friends to drive her home. One of her coworkers, an ex-drug addict, assumed the patient's behavior was due to a drug problem, and she brought the patient to the behavioral treatment unit of University Hospital. The patient was so groggy she fell asleep and did not realize where she was.

The next morning when the plaintiff woke up and realized she was in a locked psychiatric ward, she asked to be transferred to a medical ward of the hospital. She requested the physician call the other hospital and call her neurologist. Neither the physician nor hospital staff listened to the plaintiff for over 36 hours. The trial court originally dismissed the plaintiff's claim, but the appeals court over-turned that decision and plaintiff was allowed to proceed against the hospital staff and physician.

The statutory requirements for an involuntary admit were not met. There was no documentation that the patient was a danger to herself or others. There was insufficient physician examination. The staff of the behavioral unit had no right to detain the plaintiff without properly and timely obtaining appropriate release information.

In contrast, in *Mawhirt v. Ahmed* [13], 86 F.Supp.2d 81 (E.D.N.Y. 2000), plaintiff brought suit against the hospital, physicians and nurses for false imprisonment secondary to an involuntary admission and the use of restraints both physical and chemical. The difference between this case and *Brand* is that the physicians and staff had well documented the severe psychiatric state of the patient. The plaintiff was suffering from paranoid delusions that the CIA and Mafia were out to get him. Two physicians determined he was a danger to himself and others and proceeded with the appropriate procedures for the involuntary admit.

The nursing staff documented the psychotic, delusional behavior of the plaintiff as well as behavior where the plaintiff could harm himself or threaten other patients. They followed the institution's guidelines for the administration of chemical restraints and the procedures set out for the use of physical restraints. As such, the court had no difficulty in dismissing plaintiff's claims.

Documentation of the behavior necessitating the use of restraints is critical. Under no circumstances are restraints to be used for the convenience of the staff to control an unruly patient. Your institution's policy must be clear as to:

1. Under what circumstances restraints may be used;

2. How they are to be used and for how long;

3. What type of monitoring the patient will require;

4. What documentation is adequate to justify the use of these restraints; and

5. How often the physician must reorder the use of physical restraint.

Inadequate proof of the patient's condition or need for an involuntary admit was an issue in *Davis v. St. Jude Medical Center* [14]. Plaintiff was a patient on a medical unit for the treatment of pancreatitis. Approximately three weeks after this admission he was involuntarily admitted to the hospital's chemical dependency unit by a staff physician. Plaintiff repeatedly requested to be released. He even put his request in writing to the hospital's administration. He brought a habeas corpus hearing but was discharged before the hearing took place. He brought this action for **false imprisonment.** In allowing the patient to proceed with his action, the court ruled that the hospital and physicians had failed to provide the court sufficient proof of the necessity of the patient's involuntary admit or necessity of treatment. It is important to make certain that all the requirements have been met, documented and made part of the medical record.

Use of restraints is not limited to the psychiatric setting. In many hospitals and nursing homes, patients are restrained to prevent injury. **Even putting up side rails on a bed is a form of restraint.** The reasons the side rails are up should be documented in the record. If the patient refuses to allow the side rails to be put up, then have them sign a release from liability in the event of a fall. Even though it is probably not worth the paper it is written on in a court of law, it does give the patient the opportunity to appreciate the gravity of his decision to refuse the side rails. **Use of any other type of restraint, such as sheets to hold patients in wheelchairs, posey belts or any other form of physical restraint, should only be used as a last resort and must be used only as approved by hospital policy and the physician.** In all situations where possible, obtain written consent for the use of any type of restraint.

Home Care Setting

In the home care setting, it is highly recommended that home care personnel do not place patients in restraints. Home care personnel are not available for a sufficient amount of time to evaluate the patient's response to the restraints, evaluate the need for continued use of restraints, determine if the restraints are being used properly while in use, and how the patient is being monitored while in restraints. If the family puts the patient in restraints, notify the physician, obtain an order, and instruct the family of the proper care of a patient in restraints.

Against Medical Advice

Another situation that raises possible issues of false imprisonment involves patients wishing to leave the hospital against medical advice (AMA). While you may talk to the patient about the consequences of the decision to leave and you have an obligation to review with the patient all the possible complications, which could arise if they do leave AMA, you cannot prevent a competent patient from refusing treatment or leaving. This means you cannot physically bar the patient's exit. You cannot prevent the patient from getting his clothes or other personal belongings, and you cannot attempt to touch them in an effort to make them stay.

In a particularly egregious case [15], a 67-year-old man was physically prevented from leaving a nursing home for 51 days. Shortly after his nephew admitted him to the nursing home, the man attempted to leave. Nursing home employees forcibly returned him. The man continued to demand his release and made several additional attempts to leave the home. He was finally placed in a restraint chair and denied use of the phone or even access to his own clothes. The court found that the actions of the staff were in complete and utter disregard of the man's rights and were willful, reckless, and malicious in detaining him. **Where the patient is competent, he cannot be detained against his will.**

If a situation exists where the patient is clearly not competent, then a hospital may be justified in detaining the patient. In *Blackman for Blackman v. Rifkin* [16], **the patient was extremely intoxicated and had suffered head trauma.** The court ruled the hospital was justified in restraining the patient and keeping her in the hospital because the hospital could assume that the patient would have consented to treatment if she had not been in that condition. The court dismissed her false imprisonment suit. This case must be limited to its facts. While the hospital may be justified in detaining a severely intoxicated person, the hospital cannot detain a competent patient against his will.

In the case of a **minor,** the hospital can attempt to get a court order to require the family to keep the child in the hospital, but any attempt to physically restrain the child or the parent, in the absence of a court order, exposes the hospital to liability. Basically, you can talk to a patient until he refuses to listen to you, but you cannot physically prevent him from leaving.

It does not matter how noble your motives are. Patients have a right to refuse treatment. Patients also have a right to leave the hospital when they wish (unless committed through legal procedures) and to have freedom of movement. As healthcare providers, you cannot interfere with these rights without potential liability.

One other scenario may give rise to an action for false imprisonment. **When the physician has written a discharge order, the hospital cannot keep the patient until he "settles the bill."** While the patient obviously has the obligation to pay for services rendered, the hospital cannot hold him until the patient indicates how he will pay.

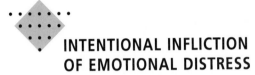

INTENTIONAL INFLICTION OF EMOTIONAL DISTRESS

In order to establish the tort of **intentional infliction of emotional distress, the plaintiff must show that the defendant's conduct is outrageous and beyond the bounds of common decency.** Insulting behavior is not enough. The actions must be egregious. One case in which the court allowed the plaintiff to proceed with his claim of intentional infliction of emotional distress is *Williams v. Payne et al.* [29]. In *Williams,* the police suspected the plaintiff of ingesting crack cocaine. Plaintiff was brought to Pontiac Osteopathic Hospital, where Dr. Brock was asked by Sheriff Payne to pump plaintiff's stomach. Dr. Brock was aware that the sheriff did not have a warrant for the search.

After placing the plaintiff in four-point restraints, Dr. Brock forcefully and over the objections of plaintiff performed the gastric lavage. Thereafter, plaintiff was involuntarily catheterized. In refusing to dismiss the claims against the hospital and doctor, the court concluded that a jury could decide whether the conduct was outrageous.

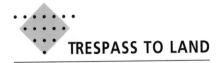

TRESPASS TO LAND

The tort of trespass to land occurs when a person, without the consent of the owner, enters onto another's land or causes anyone or anything to enter the land. Harm to the land is not required, but without harm to the land, usually only nominal damages are awarded. Trespass to land arises most often in the home health area.

In home care, the healthcare providers are guests in the patients' homes. They are there to perform necessary medical procedures and to teach, but they are still guests in the patients' homes. At anytime that a patient instructs you to leave his home, you must leave, or you are committing trespass to land. Keep in mind the landowner is authorized to use reasonable force to remove a trespasser. Even if your motives are noble in refusing to leave the property such as wanting to perform the necessary wound care for the patient's benefit, your noble intent is no defense to the tort of trespass.

QUASI-INTENTIONAL TORTS

Quasi-intentional torts include defamation, invasion of privacy, and breach of confidentiality. "Quasi" means resembling. These types of torts resemble intentional torts but are different because they are based on speech [17].

DEFAMATION

Defamation wrongfully damages the reputation of another person. **Libel** is written defamatory statements, and **slander** is spoken defamatory statements. To be liable for defamation, you must make a defamatory statement, it must be published to third parties and the speaker must have known or should have known the statements were false.

In defining what is a defamatory statement, the courts have looked to whether the statement exposed the plaintiff to public hatred, contempt, ridicule, or degradation [18]. There must be proof that there was actual harm to the reputation.

There are, however, certain statements which are considered **defamatory per se**, such as serious allegations of sexual misconduct or serious criminal behavior or allegations that the plaintiff is afflicted with a loathsome disease. Historically, loathsome diseases were considered syphilis, gonorrhea or leprosy. In modern times, allegations of positive HIV status or AIDS may well be the new loathsome disease. If these are the defamatory statements made, then the plaintiff does not need to prove actual damage to the reputation.

An example of defamation per se case is *Schlesser v. Keck* [19]. Plaintiff was a cook and caterer who tested with a false positive for syphilis when she was in the Army. She sought treatment for the false positive. Defendant was the doctor's nurse who was administering the treatments. Despite the defendant's knowledge that the tests were false positive and the defendant's knowledge that plaintiff did not have syphilis, defendant announced at a party that the plaintiff had syphilis and should not be allowed to cater or prepare food.

In addition to making a defamatory statement, there must be publication to a third person. You cannot defame someone by only telling him or her. Finally, you must know or you should have known that the statements were false.

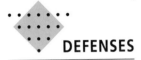

DEFENSES

Truth is an absolute defense to defamation. Even if the true statement may be damaging to the person's reputation, it is not actionable as defamation. Certain individuals such as public officials must prove actual malice on the part of the defendant before they are allowed to succeed.

In addition to the above, there may be **qualified privileges** which protect a person from a defamation suit. **One of the most common is the qualified privilege all states have enacted concerning the reporting of elder or child abuse.** As long as the report is made in good faith, the healthcare provider is protected from liability. Most states have also granted **peer review members** a qualified privilege. Such individuals must be members of a properly convened peer review committee; the committee must be duly authorized by the facility to conduct peer review; the comments made in the committee meeting and all reports of the committee must be confidential. While the member of a peer review committee may have a qualified privilege to speak freely within the confines of the committee, that privilege does not extend to speaking freely about the committee findings or proceedings to individuals not involved with the peer review committee.

The greatest liability for defamation suits results from statements made about co-employees, especially when future employers seek references. Even though a qualified privilege exists to give a good faith assessment of an employee's job performance, many businesses have opted only to verify dates of employment to avoid any allegation of defamation. **Under no circumstances should anyone give his unsolicited opinion about a former employee.**

In *Ironside v. Simi Valley Hospital* [20], Dr. Ironside sued Simi Valley Hospital for sending an unsolicited letter to the physician's new employer stating that Dr. Ironside had his privileges summarily suspended and that a report to that effect had been sent to the California Medical Board. The letter suggested the new employer check the status of Dr. Ironside's license to practice medicine with the California Medical Board. In actuality, there had been no suspension or limitation placed on Dr. Ironside's license. The letter, however, did imply that. Likewise, in *Simpkins v. District of Columbia et al.* [21], the court held that Dr. Simpkins could proceed against defendants who allegedly reported to a physician data bank that Dr. Simpkins resigned his staff privileges at the hospital during a review of the quality of care he provided.

The lesson to learn is simple. Do not talk about your fellow employees. If you are in a supervisory position, keep all comments about the quality of care rendered by the person confidential. All inquiries concerning former employees should be referred to one designated department in the facility so that standardization is maintained. Before any information is released about a former employee, have the employee's written consent to release the information as well as an agreement to release the facility from liability with regard to the information released.

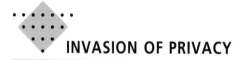

INVASION OF PRIVACY

Invasion of privacy is the tort of unjustifiably intruding upon another's right of privacy by:

1. Appropriating his or her name or likeness.
2. Unreasonably interfering with his or her seclusion.
3. Publishing private facts.
4. Placing a person in a false light.

Invasion of privacy differs from defamation. In most instances, the information is true, but it is information that a person wants to keep private. While defamation causes injury to reputation, invasion of privacy causes injury to feelings.

Appropriating Likeness and Placing Person in a False Light

In the medical setting the most common example of appropriating likeness is the use of photographs or video images of the patient without consent or exceeding the scope of the consent. For example, in *Vassiliades v. Garfinckel's, Brooks Brothers* [22], a plastic surgeon used "before" and "after" pictures of a patient in a public demonstration without the patient's consent. Another example is the use of a video of a Cesarean section not for medical teaching purposes but for inclusion in a movie that was shown publicly in movie theaters [23].

If a patient gives consent to the use of his/her likeness for teaching purposes or treatment purposes, the scope of the consent cannot be exceeded. If the patient does not give consent, then no likeness can be used at all for any reason.

Publicizing Private Facts

The most basic right of patients is to expect healthcare professionals to keep all information obtained in the treatment of the patient confidential. Every state mandates that the patient's confidentiality be maintained. Every state outlines only limited situations under which a person may release information concerning a patient without his consent.

In *Estate of Behringer v. Princeton Medical Center* [24], a successful ear, nose, and throat surgeon who practiced at the Princeton Medical Center was admitted for tests and had AIDS. No special steps were taken to protect the medical record or the patient's privacy. In fact, the physicians and nurses who cared for Dr. Behringer spoke openly about his condition to individuals who had no involvement in his care. By the time Dr. Behringer was discharged from the hospital, numerous persons in the community knew of his condition and his practice was adversely affected.

In holding that the physician could bring suit against the medical center for invasion of privacy, the court stated:

> "The information was too easily available, too titillating to disregard. All that was required was a glance at the chart, and the written words became whispers and the whispers became roars" [25].

The whispers should never have taken place. Likewise, in *Doe v. Methodist Hospital* [26], a patient's HIV status was openly discussed with individuals not involved with his care. Plaintiff suffered a heart attack and was taken to the hospital by paramedics. He disclosed to the paramedics his HIV status. They noted this on their report, which became part of the medical record. One of plaintiff's coworkers called his wife, who was a nurse at the hospital, and she reviewed the patient's records and told her husband the plaintiff's HIV status. While the Indiana Supreme Court ruled that Indiana does not recognize the tort of invasion of privacy, the suit was allowed to proceed under other causes of actions.

Disclosing confidential patient information may lead to lawsuits under a number of legal theories of liability, including **breach of contract, breach of confidence, negligence, intentional infliction of emotional distress and defamation.**

Even disclosing information to other healthcare professionals may lead to a lawsuit. In *Saur v. Probes* [27], plaintiff's wife attempted to have plaintiff involuntarily committed for psychiatric treatment. She went to court and the court appointed a psychiatrist to examine the plaintiff. The court-appointed psychiatrist contacted the defendant, who had been plaintiff's treating physician for several months. The two physicians discussed the plaintiff's medical condition. The plaintiff filed this action against his treating psychiatrist alleging that the psychiatrist disclosed confidential information obtained during the course of treatment without patient's permission. The lower court dismissed the plaintiff's case, but the higher court reversed, finding that plaintiff was entitled to have his case heard before a jury to decide whether the disclosure was appropriate. Whether this plaintiff ultimately wins is not the issue. The issue is the court allowed the case to proceed to the jury.

Being a healthcare provider and working in a medical facility do not give you the right to unlimited access to all patients' medical records. You are allowed in law only to view and use the medical records of the patients you are treating.

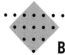

BREACH OF CONFIDENTIALITY

The computer age is creating even more problems for **breach of confidentiality**. While allowing practitioners to have easier access to their patient records and allowing information to be relayed more quickly, computerized medical records allow too many people acess. A case in point was filed in 1997 in Fulton County, Georgia. In *Ruocco v. Emory Hospital* [28], plaintiff filed a lawsuit alleging invasion of privacy, negligent maintenance of records, negligent supervision, intentional infliction of emotional distress and defamation.

Plaintiff was a nurse employed by Emory Hospital who was taking part in a hepatitis study. She received injections as part of the study. When she missed several weeks of work, one of the doctors in the study accessed her electronic medical record without the plaintiff's permission. Although he was not plaintiff's treating physician, he accessed the records by claiming to be her physician. He was not. He did not tell the plaintiff he accessed the records and, in fact, in his deposition stated he never intended to tell her. Plaintiff learned of the unauthorized access when she accessed her own records and saw that someone had accessed her records without her consent. (As of this writing, no disposition to this case is known.)

The concern over electronic access to medical records has been increasing. In 1996, Congress enacted the **Health Insurance Portability and Accountability Act of 1996,** calling for regulations to establish criteria for a federal standard in authorizing the release of medical information, and in February 2000 the final rules to establish the federal criteria were published by the U.S. Department of Health and Human Services.

Whether a healthcare provider has access to the traditional written medical record or to the new computerized records, the responsibility to keep the information confidential does not change. **Any information that a healthcare provider learns while taking care of a patient is confidential, even if it does not relate directly to the treatment of the patient.**

The issue of confidentiality is both a legal and ethical issue. The code of ethics of allied health personnel must emphasize that the healthcare professional must safeguard the patient's right to privacy by judiciously protecting confidential information. Many other groups, such as the Hospice Association of America, American Nurses Association, National League for Nursing, and the American Hospital Association, recognize as a basic right of patients the confidentiality of the assessments, treatment, and information contained in the patient's medical records.

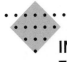

INTENTIONAL AND QUASI-INTENTIONAL TORTS AND INSURANCE POLICIES

Even though intentional torts have historically been covered under medical malpractice policies, many insurers are writing exclusions from coverage. This is especially true if the tort alleged involves sexual misconduct. As a healthcare provider, know what your policy covers and what it does not.

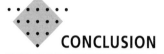

CONCLUSION

The performance of day-to-day patient care and treatment gives rise to potential liability for intentional and quasi-intentional torts. That liability can be avoided if you always have your patient's consent to perform specific procedures and do not exceed that consent. Always maintain your patient's confidentiality, speaking only to those individuals who are actively involved in the patient's care. Understand that your patient has an absolute right to refuse treatment and that your ability to change a person's mind is limited to your verbal skills only. It is not true that every patient is a potential plaintiff. But a patient can be turned into a plaintiff if you do not exercise good nursing judgment or do not have respect for your patient's rights, privacy and freedom.

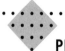

PERTINENT POINTS

1. In order to be successful in pursuing a lawsuit for an intentional tort, the plaintiff must prove that the defendant had the requisite intent, that the injury resulted from the defendant's action, and that no defense was present.

2. If a defendant can prove that the plaintiff gave consent, then no intentional tort has been committed.

3. The defendant must stay within the boundaries of the consent given by the plaintiff. If the scope of the consent is exceeded, then it is as though there was no consent.

4. Forcing treatment on an unwilling patient is assault and battery.

5. If procedures for involuntary admits are not followed, then false imprisonment may occur. If force is used to detain a patient, then false imprisonment has occurred. No matter how noble a healthcare worker's motives may be, he has no right

to forcibly detain a patient who is competent and not a danger to himself or others.

6. Invasion of privacy is likely to occur in the healthcare setting if healthcare professionals do not maintain the confidentiality of patient records.

7. All patients have the right to expect that heathcare professionals will maintain the confidentiality of medical records.

8. Trespass to land occurs most often in the home health setting.

STUDY QUESTIONS

1. Define an intentional tort and quasi-intentional tort.

2. Give examples of and be able to discuss the following torts:

   a. Assault

   b. Battery

   c. False imprisonment

   d. Defamation

   e. Invasion of privacy

   f. Intentional infliction of emotional distress

   g. Trespass to land.

3. Discuss the intent required to commit an intentional tort.

4. Discuss what effect consent has in defending an intentional tort.

5. Discuss a recent case with the class involving an intentional or quasi-intentional tort in your area.

REFERENCES

1. Schloendorff v. Society of New York Hospital, 211 N.Y. 125 (1914).
2. Pizzaloto v. Wilson, 437 So.2d 859 (La. 1983).
3. Guin v. Sison, 552 So.2d 60 (La.App. 3rd Cir. 1989).
4. Montgomery v. Bazaz-Shegal, 742 A.2d 1125 (Pa.Super. 1999).

5. Roberson v. Provident House, 576 So.2d 992 (La. 1991).

6. O'Brien v. Cunard Steamship Co., 154 Mass. 272, 28 N.E. 266 (1881).

7. Novak v. Cobb County Kennestone Hospital Authority, slip opinion no. 94-8403 (11th Cir. 1996).

8. DiLeo v. Nugent, 592 A.2d 1126 (Md.App. 1991).

9. Smith v. St. Paul Fire and Marine Insurance Co., 353 N.W.2d 130 (Minn. 1984).

10. St. Paul Fire and Marine Insurance Co. v. Asbury, 720 P.3d 540 (Ariz. 1986).

11. St. Paul Fire and Marine Insurance Co. v. Shernow, 222 Conn. 823 (1992).

12. Brand v. University Hospital, 525 S.E.2d 374 (Ga.App. 1999).

13. Mawhirt v. Ahmed, 86 F.Supp.2d 81 (E.D.N.Y. 2000).

14. Davis v. St. Jude Medical Center, 645 So.2d 771 (La.App. 5th Cir. 1994).

15. Big Town Nursing Home, Inc. v. New, 461 S.W.2d 195 (Tex.Civ.App. 1970).

16. Blackman for Blackman v. Rifkin, 759 P.2d 54 (Colo.App. 1988, cert. denied 1989).

17. Aiken T. (Ed.) (2002). *Legal, ethical and political issues in nursing* (2nd ed). Philadelphia: F.A. Davis Company.

18. Phipps v. Clark Oil and Refining Corp., 408 N.W.2d 569, 573 (Minn. 1987).

19. Schlesser v. Keck, 271 P.2d 588 (Cal.App. 1954).

20. Ironside v. Simi Valley Hospital, slip opinion no. 95-6336 (6th Cir. 1996).

21. Simpkins v. District of Columbia et al., slip opinion no. 94-5243 (D.C. Cir. 1997).

22. Vassiliades v. Garfinckel's, Brooks Brothers, 492 A.2d 580 (D.C.App. 1985).

23. Feeney v. Young, 191 A.D. 501 (1920).

24. Estate of Behringer v. Princeton Medical Center, 592 A.2d 1251 (N.J.Super. 1991).

25. Id. At 1273.

26. Doe v. Methodist Hospital, 639 N.E.2d 683 (Ind.App. 1Dist. 1994); 690 N.E.2d 681 (Ind. 1997).

27. Saur v. Probes, 476 N.W.2d 496 (Mich.App. 1991).

28. Ruocco v. Emory Hospital, no. 97-VS-0132401.

29. Williams v. Payne et al., 73 F.Supp.2d 785 (E.D.Mich. 1999).

3

Professional Liability Insurance

M. LEE LEPPANEN, RN, JD

▶ **Key Chapter Concepts**

Aggregate Limit
Claims-Made Policy
Endorsement
Excess Coverage
Exclusions
Insuring Agreement or Clause
Occurrence Policy
Prior Acts Coverage
Tail Coverage

▶ **Objectives**

At the conclusion of this chapter, the reader will have a better understanding of:

1. The basic professional liability insurance terms and concepts.

2. The necessity for professional liability insurance for independent contractors and employed healthcare professionals.

3. The employer's liability policy exclusions and their effect on individual employee liability.

4. The typical components of a professional liability policy.

LIABILITY INSURANCE IN GENERAL

The overall purpose of liability insurance is to spread the risk of economic loss among members of a group who have a commonly shared risk. A small fee, a **premium**, is contributed by each insured member and pooled by the insurer into a fund. An injured party then uses this fund to pay for claims against any of the members. This avoids the often economically devastating costs associated with defending yourself against such claims. Nonmeritorious claims can be just as costly to defend as meritorious ones.

▶ Case Scenario

A patient was treated as an outpatient at a medical facility and was prescribed a sulfa drug. The patient was allergic to sulfa drugs, a fact that was noted in the written medical record. However, the medical records technician did not transcribe the allergy note into the computerized patient record. Upon discharge from the facility, the nurse failed to check the written record. The pharmacist who dispensed the drug did not note the allergy. After taking one dose of the sulfa drug, the patient had a severe allergic reaction which ultimately led to her death. The patient's family sued the pharmacist and the facility for the negligence of the nurse and the medical records technician. If the claim against the technician was made after the technician left the facility's employ, did the facility's liability insurance provide coverage to defend the technician? You will learn the answer at the end of this chapter.

Individually, the prime objective is to protect your assets in the event of a judgment or settlement in favor of the claimant. Some professionals do not see a need to obtain liability insurance because they feel that they do not have that much to protect. They believe they are "judgment-free," so that even if a claim against them is successful, they have little that the claimant could collect. This assumption is erroneous. First, although one has few assets now, it is reasonable to assume that most professionals will have assets worth protecting in the future. If a claimant secures a judgment against you, that judgment stands and can be enforced at a later time when your assets may have increased substantially. Even if you have insurance by that time, it will not provide coverage. Besides losing a substantial portion of your assets, there can be worse ramifications, such as bankruptcy.

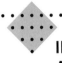

INDEPENDENT CONTRACTORS AND EMPLOYED PROFESSIONALS: THE NEED FOR AN INDIVIDUAL POLICY

A healthcare professional who is an independent contractor most definitely should obtain liability insurance. An **independent contractor** is a person who is self-employed and who enters into contracts to provide professional services to various entities such as hospitals, doctors' offices and/or individual clients. Generally, these entities will have no liability for the acts or omissions of an independent contractor unless the entity can be found directly liable, as discussed in the next section [1]. Most of these contracting entities will require that the independent contractor show evidence of current liability coverage. Even if not required, securing coverage to protect your assets is exceedingly important as discussed earlier.

The employed practitioner, even though provided coverage by the employer, should also obtain a professional liability policy. To understand why this is so, first consider employers liability policies.

EMPLOYERS LIABILITY POLICIES

An employer such as a hospital or doctor's office obtains professional liability insurance to protect its own interests. With respect to its liability for the negligent acts of an employee or independent contractor, the employer seeks to protect itself against claims that fall generally under two theories of liability. First, the employer can have a claim filed against it charging that it is directly liable for the injury of claimant caused by an employee or independent contractor. Under this theory, the claimant commonly alleges the following:

1. When the employer hired the employee, the employer failed its duty to ascertain that the employee had the necessary qualifications and capability to render safe care.

2. The employer failed to adequately supervise the employee.

3. The employer failed to provide the employee with the proper training required to render safe care.

The employer can also be sued under a theory of **vicarious liability,** wherein the acts or omissions of the employee are imputed to the employer, so that the employer can be found liable for them [23].

Coverage and Exclusions

Generally, the liability policies that employers obtain in order to protect them in the event of such allegations provide liability for the employee as well. The employer's policy spells out specifically those acts of the employee that are covered and acts that are excluded from coverage. Commonly, the employee is covered under the employer's policy for a negligent act only if it was performed within the scope of the employee's duties.

Acts that often are specifically excluded are those such as **libel** or **slander** and **intentional acts** which an employee intends or expects will result in an injury. If a claim is made against an employer for the acts of an employee that are covered by the policy, then the insurer has a duty to defend the employee as well as the employer. The insurer's duty to defend generally includes, for example, providing legal counsel to represent the employer and employee in negotiations with the claimant, representation in court proceedings, filing court documents, investigating the alleged incident and advising the client regarding case strategy. However, see the discussion below regarding conflicts of interest between employer and employee that can arise in such situations.

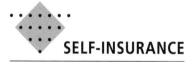

SELF-INSURANCE

Some healthcare institutions elect to **self-insure** in accordance with state laws. No insurance policy may be obtained, but the employer must provide evidence that it has sufficient funds set aside to satisfy a successful claim. Whether the employer self-insures or purchases coverage, keep in mind that the employer is looking out for the employer's own interests first and foremost. This is particularly true, however, where the employer self-insures, because then the employer has more control in the defense of a claim.

EMPLOYED PROFESSIONALS: THE NEED FOR THEIR OWN PROFESSIONAL LIABILITY INSURANCE

There are a host of reasons why the prudent employed professional obtains his own professional liability insurance. The reasons for insurance are as follows:

Acts Not Covered

The employer's policy does not provide coverage for certain acts of the employee. For example, a medical assistant makes a remark to a coworker about a client that the client overhears and reasonably perceives to be defamatory. The employer's policy will probably not provide coverage for this incident, and the employee will have to defend against a lawsuit. Even if the employee successfully defends against such allegations, the costs of doing so can be substantial. Policies are available to individuals that provide coverage for many acts that are not covered under an employer's policy.

Limits of Policy Exceeded

An employer's policy, as with any insurance policy, has limits as to how much the insurer pays. If an incident involves multiple alleged acts of negligence and/or claimants, it is possible for the employer's policy limits to be exceeded. In that case, the employee may be responsible for financing all or part of the defense.

Mergers and Closures of Physicians' Offices and Healthcare Facilities

In today's healthcare environment, the "urge to merge" has resulted in complex restructuring schemes. The terms of agreement between two merging entities can result in changes in the employer's liability insurance coverage. Depending on the terms of the employer's policy and the date of an incident involving the employees, the latter can find they are without employer coverage for a given incident that was covered under their employer's policy prior to the merger. A worse scenario can occur when a facility closes. The employer may not have purchased a policy to cover claims that are made after the closure, and the employee may therefore be left "bare," meaning that the insurance company will not pay for defense costs and money awards.

Conflict Between Employer and Employee as to Their Respective Positions Regarding an Incident

In a given incident that results in a claim, the employer may not agree with the employee's view of that incident. For example, the employer takes the position that in a given incident the employee was not acting within the scope of his duties. If the employer proves this to be true, the employer's insurer (or especially the employer if self-insured) has no duty to assist in the employee's defense [4]. At the very least, the fact that the employee and the employer disagree as to the facts of an incident can create problems in the defense strategy of the insurer's attorney. It is far better to have your own policy and your own attorney whose loyalty will be only to you, the employee.

Disagreement Between Employer and Employee Regarding Proposed Settlements

The employer may wish to settle a claim rather than defend a lawsuit for any number of reasons. The employer may wish to limit unfavorable publicity, or it may not wish to devote the personnel time and other resources necessary to defend the case. The employer's insurer may concur if the claimant appears to have at least a 50% chance of winning at trial. It may be more cost effective for the insurer to settle the case rather than risk going to trial and have a jury award of a substantially higher amount. Even though the employee may have strong feelings regarding the lack of negligence on his part in an incident, the best interests of the employee are not primary; those of the employer are. If the employer is self-insured, the focus of loyalty is obvious [5].

Conflict Between Multiple Employees Regarding an Incident

Many incidents involve multiple employees. In such situations, the claimant sues everyone connected with the incident: the employer, supervisors and employees. Attorneys do not want the clients to later accuse them of negligent handling of their case. The potential for disagreement regarding essential facts of an incident can put an individual at odds with not only supervisors, but with coworkers who, after all, are trying to protect themselves. Your own insurer and attorney have loyalty only to you and will formulate a defense strategy that is in your best interest rather than one which must take into account the positions of your coworkers.

Cost

A professional liability policy for an employed health occupation professional is generally quite inexpensive. Such policies can be purchased for an annual premium that is under $100.00. At such a low cost and given the protection the policy affords, the professional should not practice without it.

Peace of Mind

The benefit of knowing that you have someone on your side if you are ever involved in a claim against you is priceless. An attorney is provided to assist you in your defense. Also, if a judgment is awarded against you, the insurance company pays the money award to the plaintiff. It will not come "out of your pocket."

APPLYING FOR PROFESSIONAL LIABILITY INSURANCE

An insurer will take into account an individual practitioner's situation in recommending policy provisions and limits of coverage. An applicant must be thorough and honest in providing information to the insurance representative. If you are an independent contractor, inform the representative of the details of your practice including, but not limited to, the following:

1. **What services do you provide?** Inform the representative about not only what your typical day-to-day duties are, but those services that you may provide on rare occasions, as well as those that you do not provide now but are considering in the future. This prevents denial of coverage by your insurer due to your concealment or misrepresentation if an incident occurs while performing a service you did not previously mention [6]. Also, the representative will take your specific occupation into account. For example, some services that are provided by a physical therapist have a higher incidence of related claims than most of those provided by a medical records technician.

2. **What type of clients do you serve?** For example, are the clients frail, elderly, children or disabled?

3. **Do you employ or supervise others, even if only occasionally?**

4. **Are you supervised and by whom?** Supervision may affect the independent contractor status.

5. **Are you in compliance with all licensing requirements, if required in your state?**

6. **Have you ever had a lawsuit filed against you?**

7. **Have you ever had a complaint made against you to the disciplinary body that governs your practice?**

8. **Are there any incidents that have occurred in the past that could possibly give rise to a future claim?**

COMPONENTS OF A TYPICAL PROFESSIONAL LIABILITY POLICY

A practitioner's liability insurance policy will be tailored to fit a specific type of practice (Box 3–1). However, the provisions typically include the following.

At the beginning of the policy form, there is usually a statement that it is a **claims-made** or an **occurrence** policy. A **claims-made trigger** means that coverage is provided for any claim made while the policy is in force.

BOX 3–1 • TYPES OF POLICIES

- *Claims-Made*–A type of professional liability insurance policy that covers injuries only if the injury occurs in the policy period and the claim is reported to the insurance company during the policy period or during the "tail."
- *Occurrence*–Professional liability insurance policy that covers injuries that occur during the period covered by the policy even though they may be reported outside the policy period.
- *Tail Coverage*–An uninterrupted extension of the insurance policy period, also known as the extended reporting endorsement.
- *Umbrella Coverage*–Is purchased in addition to a basic liability policy. It provides additional amount limits and/or adds coverage for events not covered in the basic policy.

For example, you purchase a claims-made policy with coverage from September 1, 2000, through August 31, 2001, but at the end of that term you decide not to renew because you are no longer going to work. If a claim is made against you on July 1, 2001, coverage applies. However, if the incident giving rise to the claim occurred during the policy period on March 1, 2001, but the claim was not made against you until November 1, 2001, there is usually no coverage.

Some policies provide that if you notify your insurer, prior to the expiration of the policy, of an incident that you believe could evolve into a claim, then coverage is provided. Also, many policies provide, at no extra charge, a 60-day extension following expiration of the policy during which the insurer will defend you in a claim filed during that 60-day period. If neither of these two modifications for coverage exist, then you should consider purchasing **"tail"** coverage. (Insurers should check the applicable statutes of limitations for filing lawsuits in their states.)

Tail Coverage

Tail coverage is a special policy that extends the coverage provided in the original policy for an agreed upon period of time. If in the above example you purchased a tail to extend coverage until August 31, 2006, and a claim was made on June 1, 2005, coverage applies.

Prior Acts Coverage

Another concern with claims-made policies is that they generally do not cover "prior acts." **Prior acts** are those incidents that occurred prior to the beginning effective date of the policy. Prior acts coverage can be purchased for an additional premium. The insurer issues *"prior acts"* coverage going back for a certain period of time. The insurer requires that the professional provide the following information:

1. Services that were provided;
2. Whether the professional was employed or self-employed; and
3. Details regarding any incident that the professional believes might possibly evolve into a claim.

Not divulging such information can result in the insurer having no obligation to provide a defense for any claim related to the nondivulged incident.

Occurrence Policy

An **"occurrence"** policy provides coverage for an incident that occurs during the policy period, regardless of when the claim is made. For example, you purchase an occurrence policy with coverage from September 1, 2000, through August 31, 2005, but then decide not to renew the policy. If a claim is made on May 1, 2006, based on an incident that occurred during the policy period, coverage applies. You would not, however, have coverage for any incident that occurred before the beginning effective date of the policy period unless you purchased *prior acts coverage.*

Occurrence-type coverage offers the safest protection because you usually know if an incident may trigger a claim. Insurers are increasingly omitting occurrence policies in favor of **claims-made policies.** This is probably because the period of time for which an insurer must be concerned about a claim can be definitely determined.

Medical facilities usually obtain occurrence policies [7]. Under that type of policy, if you no longer work for that employer, the employer and you still have coverage for an incident that occurred while you were employed. However, if the employer has a claims-made policy, then your coverage depends on the policy provisions. The importance of knowing the provisions in your employer's policy is evident because you should know whether or not to consider purchasing tail coverage.

Declarations Page

Frequently called the **"dec"** page in insurance jargon, this is where the policy lists the name(s) of the person or institution insured. The **"aggregate"** amount is the total amount that the insurer pays during the policy period, usually one year, regardless of the number of incidents, claims, claimants or defendants. For example, the employer's policy declarations page provides for $3 million of aggregate coverage.

Assume that the incident described in the example above has occurred and that $1 million has been used in providing a defense for that incident. Then $2 million of coverage remains for the balance of the policy period. This may seem like a large amount, but it can easily be exhausted if the institution has several serious incidents that occur during a policy period, and it provides another reason why you should consider obtaining a personal policy.

The declarations page also notes the dates indicating the period of time for which coverage is provided and the premium charged.

In the case of an employer, it also lists the categories of employees that are covered. Additionally, the declarations page will spell out the **limits of liability.**

There are two types of limitations on liability: per **incident** or **occurrence** and **aggregate,** and there are dollar amounts noted for each type. **Per incident** (in a health professional's policy it is usually called a **medical incident**) amounts show the maximum amount that the insurer will pay for defending a claim that arises from a single incident.

For example, the declarations page shows "$1,000,000 per incident." This means that the insurer pays up to that amount only, regardless of the number of claimants or insured involved. Suppose that three radiology technicians are negligent in transferring a patient from the x-ray table to the gurney and the patient falls, sustaining a serious head injury. The patient sues for the injury. The spouse sues for loss of consortium, and their child sues for loss of society and companionship. An employer's policy having $1 million per incident coverage pays for the defense of the employer. This amount is also used to pay for the defense of the radiology technicians. This illustrates once more the importance of healthcare employees purchasing their own liability policies.

The practitioner may also want to consider additional liability protection by purchasing an "umbrella" policy. The maximum amount payable under a basic liability policy may become exhausted, for example, where there have been multiple claims. An umbrella policy provides coverage beyond the amount limits of the basic policy. It may also provide coverage for events that were excluded from coverage under a basic policy. For example, an umbrella policy may be written to provide coverage for allegations of defamation where there is no such coverage under the basic policy. The cost of an umbrella policy is determined by the amount of coverage desired and the particular events covered. The practitioner should discuss his or her particular situation with an insurance representative to determine whether the addition of an umbrella policy is appropriate.

INDIVIDUAL PROFESSIONAL LIABILITY POLICIES

Regarding individual professional liability policies, most practitioners obtain policies with limits of $1 million per medical incident and $3 million in the aggregate. However, insurers offer higher limits and practitioners should discuss their particular practices with a representative to determine what coverage level is appropriate.

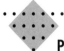

POLICY PROVISIONS

Sometimes called the **"policy jacket,"** this section sets forth the generic provisions that are found in most policies of the same type (Box 3–2). The provisions are usually separated into separate sections and generally include the following items:

Statement of the Agreement

This statement is often called the **"insuring agreement"** or **"insuring clause"** and states the agreement between the insurer and the insured as to what coverage is provided. The clause briefly states what type of claims (e.g., damages due to injury) the insurer is obligated to pay and under what conditions (e.g., injury due to acts or omissions of the insured) while the policy is in force.

BOX 3–2 • POLICY PROVISIONS

- Statement of agreement
- Exclusions
- Duties and cooperation of insured
- Definitions
- Nonrenewal or cancellation
- Right to defend or settle
- Other insurance

Exclusions

This section enumerates in detail all of the circumstances for which coverage is provided. Typical examples include, but are not limited to:

1. *Claims* alleging defamation, sexual assault or discrimination;
2. *Claims* resulting from an incident that occurred prior to the effective date of the policy;
3. *Claims* resulting from an injury the insured either expected or intended;
4. *Claims* arising under any contract the insured has wherein the insured agreed to assume the liability of others; and
5. *Claims* arising out of the commission of a criminal act.

Duties and Cooperation of Insured

This section lists the duties and required cooperation of the insured in the event of a claim and/or incident. It states how soon after a claim the insured must notify the insurer. Sometimes this is a specific number of days, but commonly the time frame may be quite vague, saying "as soon as practicable." There may or may not be a requirement that the notification be in writing. However, the prudent professional sends written notification by certified mail with a return receipt requested. The cooperation of the insured usually includes assisting in securing and giving evidence, attending hearings and trials, helping secure the attendance of witnesses and assisting in the enforcement of any right of "contribution" or "indemnity" which the insured has against others.

A right of **contribution** arises when there are others who, although not named in a claim, bear at least some responsibility for the incident. The insured, if found liable, has a right in some states to seek contribution from others based on a percentage of their responsibility in causing the incident. A right to **indemnification** arises under similar circumstances except that the insured contends that some other person was totally responsible for the incident and that, therefore, that other person should reimburse the insured for the entire amount he or she has paid [8].

Definitions

All of the words in a policy that are considered to be insurance terms that the average person may not know are defined. Also defined are those terms that the insurer wants to be sure will be construed by the courts in a certain way if a question of coverage arises. Such words as **"medical incidents," "claim," "injury"** and even **"you"** are usually defined.

Nonrenewal or Cancellation

In this section, the conditions under which the insurer can elect to not renew or to cancel the policy are described. Usually, the insurer does not need to have a reason. However, there are generally requirements for providing notice to the insured. Typically, if the insurer is not renewing the policy, it must notify the insured in writing at least 30 days prior to the policy expiration date. If the insurer plans to cancel the policy, most policy provisions state that it must provide written notice at least 10 days prior to cancellation for nonpayment of the premium and at least 30 days prior to cancellation if for any other reason.

Right to Defend or Settle

The insurer states in this section its duty to defend claims as well as its right to do so, even if the facts indicate that the claim has no merit or appears to be fraudulent [9]. This is the section where the insurer may also state that it has a right to settle a claim, if it determines that settlement is appropriate, without the permission of the insured. One reason the insurer may offer settlement to a claimant is that it believes the claimant has a plausible claim that may result in a high jury award if litigated. Also, the claimant may offer to settle for an amount that the insurer believes is less than the claimant might receive if he or she prevails at trial. In either case, the insured may have little or no input in the decision, even if the insured believes that he or she has done nothing wrong.

Other Insurance

Typically, this section addresses how the payment of claims is affected if there is other insurance available to pay a given claim. This situation arises where, for example, there is an employer's policy and a second (e.g., professional's individual) policy that provide coverage for a single medical incident. The employer's policy may state it will only apply after the second policy's limits have been paid. The amount the insurer is obligated to pay after the second policy has been paid is called **"excess coverage."** If the second policy has the same provision, so that both policies are "excess coverage," then the two insurers will generally share equally in the total amount paid to defend the claim [10].

Expenses of Defending a Claim

Some policies provide that the expenses (e.g., attorneys fees, expert witness fees, etc.) are included in the limits of liability amounts. This results in reducing the amount available to pay the claimant's damages, regardless of whether those damages are determined by settlement or mediation/arbitration. Other policies provide that expenses are paid over and above whatever the claimant actually receives.

Premium Payments

Usually, this section does not provide information regarding the time, method or amount of the premium but states that the rates are in accordance with those in effect at the time and that the premiums are payable when they become due. As discussed earlier, an insurer generally cannot cancel a policy for default in premium payment until it has provided to the insured a timely notice of premium due and intent to cancel prior to cancellation.

Endorsements

The policy usually contains added provisions that delete or modify the coverage provided in the standard provisions or "policy jacket" part of the policy. These provisions, sometimes called **"riders,"** address items that apply to the insured's specific situation. For example, there may be a provision that the insurer pays for expenses resulting from the insured being the victim of an assault while he or she is at work and possibly while traveling to and from work. The insurer may provide coverage for claims due to defamation or other nonmedical incidents. The insurer may grant an option to the insured to extend liability coverage (i.e., purchase "tail" coverage) upon termination of the policy.

PRIOR TO PURCHASING A POLICY

The time to determine what protection a professional liability policy provides is prior to its purchase, not when a claim is filed. Prior to purchase, a professional should obtain a sample policy and then discuss any questions with the insurance agent. When the policy is issued, the professional should read the entire policy to be sure that it provides the coverage discussed with the agent. Even the most proficient and careful practitioner can be sued when there is no wrongful act or neglect on his part. Having a liability policy ensures that the professional is not subject to the possible economic disaster than can result in defending a claim or having a judgment awarded against him.

CONCLUSION

Let us return to the case scenario at the beginning of this chapter. The scenario is based on a similar set of facts in a real case where the medical records technician was, indeed, sued [11]. As you learned in this chapter, whether or not the employer's liability policy provides a defense for the technician depends on the type of policy the employer has. If it is an occurrence policy, then the technician is covered, even though the technician is no longer employed at the facility, because the incident occurred during the policy period. However, if it is a claims-made policy, then coverage depends on whether there are any policy provisions that allow coverage. If the technician wisely obtained an individual policy, taking into account the possible need for tail coverage, then the professional has coverage.

PERTINENT POINTS

1. Health occupation professionals should obtain their own professional liability insurance whether they are practicing as an independent contractor or an employee of a facility.

2. Health occupation professionals should have a comprehensive understanding of all aspects of a professional liability policy prior to its purchase.

3. Health occupation employees should be knowledgeable of the provisions in their employer's liability policy.

4. The exclusions in an employer's liability policy can result in no coverage for specific incidents involving employees or give rise to conflicts of interest between employer and employee.

5. There are two types of professional liability insurance policies: claims-made and occurrence.

STUDY QUESTIONS

1. What is the purpose of professional liability insurance?

2. How does an independent contractor differ from an employee?

3. What is vicarious liability?

4. How is self-insurance by employers different from buying an insurance policy?

5. Why do you as a healthcare professional need professional liability insurance? (List and discuss nine reasons.)

6. If you are an independent contractor, list and discuss the topics you should discuss with an insurance representative when applying for professional liability insurance.

7. What are the components of a typical professional liability policy? List and discuss them.

8. How does a claims-made policy differ from an occurrence policy?

9. Discuss the typical policy provisions found in individual professional policies.

10. What should you do prior to purchasing a professional liability policy?

REFERENCES

1. Prosser, W. (1971). *Handbook of the law of torts* (pp. 468–475). St. Paul: West Publishing Co.
2. Id. at 458-459.
3. Smith, J. W. (1998) *Hospital liability.* New York: Law Journal Seminars-Press. Section 5.01 (7).
4. Glannon, J. W. (1995). *The law of torts* (pp. 375–378). Boston: Little, Brown & Co.
5. Smith, supra at section 5.02 (3).
6. Dobbyn, J. F. (1989). *Insurance law* (pp. 152–160). St. Paul: West Publishing Co.
7. Smith, supra at section 5.01 (3).
8. Prosser, supra at 305-313.
9. Smith, supra at section 5.01 (6).
10. Id. at section 5.01 (7).
11. Harris County Hospital District v. Estrada, 872 S.W.2d 729 (Texas 1993).

4

Informed Consent Issues

MARY POWERS ANTOINE, RN, JD

▶ Objectives

Upon completion of this chapter, the reader will have a better understanding of:

1. The healthcare worker's obligations regarding the informed consent process.

2. Who may give consent on behalf of the patient when the patient is unable to do so.

3. What kinds of circumstances may give rise to special rules regarding informed consent.

 ## BATTERY/NEGLIGENCE

The law regarding informed consent has been evolving since the early part of the 20th century. In 1914, Justice Cardozo made the now famous statement quoted in Box 4–1 [1]. This statement has served as the foundation for the principles of informed consent as

▶ Case Scenario

Mrs. Richards is an elderly woman who is in the advanced stages of Alzheimer's disease. Her husband has been noticing that lately she has had bloody stools. On Tuesday January 9, Mrs. Richards comes to the hospital for a colonoscopy procedure to rule out colon cancer. Susan White is the radiology technician working in the radiology department that day. When Mrs. Richards arrives with her husband, Susan escorts them into a waiting area. Susan notes that the consent form for the procedure has not been signed. Susan hands the form to Mrs. Richards and asks her to sign it. Mr. Richards takes the form out of her hands and says that he has always made the decisions in their family and that he is going to sign the form. He then proceeds to ask Susan to explain the potential risks and side effects of the procedure. She attempts to answer his questions as best she can. Susan is uncertain whether Mr. Richards should sign the consent form, but she lets him do it. The principles of informed consent discussed in this chapter will help us analyze Susan's dilemma.

we know them today. Following this case, the law defined unwanted or unauthorized medical treatment as a battery. A battery occurs whenever one person intentionally touches another without permission. Theoretically, a claim for battery may also arise if the patient consents to a particular procedure and the physician goes beyond the scope of that consent. A battery may also occur if the physician performs a different procedure for which consent was not obtained.

BOX 4–1 • FOUNDATION FOR INFORMED CONSENT DOCTRINE

"Every competent adult has the right to make decisions regarding his or her body and medical care. This right may only be infringed upon in exceptional circumstances."

Justice Cardozo

As the law regarding informed consent began to develop, courts slowly moved away from classifying lack of informed consent as a battery. Instead, courts have ruled that informed consent more properly belongs in the area of negligence law, the classification of medical malpractice. In the leading case of *Cobbs v. Grant* [2], the California Supreme Court explained that battery should be reserved for those circumstances where no consent at all had been obtained. Where the issue is failure to disclose a particular risk, the lawsuit is more appropriately one for negligence.

As courts across the country began to rule on battery and negligence cases, the concept of "informed consent" became more defined. The individual's fundamental right to control what happens to his or her body cannot be taken away except in exceptional circumstances. This right includes the right to decide whether to accept or reject proposed medical treatment. The physician has both a legal and an ethical obligation to obtain the patient's consent, or the consent of the patient's legal representative, before performing any kind of significant medical treatment.

OBLIGATION TO OBTAIN INFORMED CONSENT

The obligation to obtain informed consent ordinarily resides with the physician who is performing the procedure. Thus, when a patient is about to undergo surgery, the physician should be the one to explain the risks and benefits of the proposed surgery. When other healthcare providers with independent authority are performing the procedure, such as a nurse practitioner or physician's assistant, the duty to obtain informed consent may fall upon those individuals. Whenever the procedure is being performed or overseen by a physician, the primary responsibility for the informed consent falls upon the physician even though there may be other people involved in the care. For example, when a procedure involves others (such as technicians or nurses), these individuals should not take it upon themselves to explain the risks and benefits of the procedure to the patient. However, the nurse or technician should bring problems and misunderstandings to the attention of the physician or a supervisor. Furthermore, the nurse or technician may serve as a witness when the patient signs the consent form. Most healthcare facilities have specific policies relating to informed consent obligations. You should become familiar with your employer's rules regarding the informed consent process.

DISCLOSURE REQUIREMENTS

Before performing medical treatment, the physician has the duty to disclose to the patient enough information to enable the patient to make an informed decision whether to accept or reject the treatment (see Box 4–2). Courts have generally agreed that the patient must be advised about the nature and purpose of the treatment, the risks and consequences of the treatment, the alternative courses of treatment, and the consequences of refusing the recommended treatment. The physician should explain the type of treatment involved and the kinds of results that are being sought. Failure to explain to the patient the relevant risks of a treatment or procedure or the extent of the risks involved is the most common source of liability for lack of informed consent. Ordinarily, the physician is expected to disclose the most frequently experienced side effects of the proposed treatment, as well as the most significant ones. Further, the physician should explain the anticipated consequences for refusing to undergo the recommended treatment. (For example, refusal to undergo a rectal exam or a colonoscopy may result in colon cancer going undetected.) In order to obtain true consent, the patient must be given the opportunity to evaluate all the options available. In order to do this, the patient must also be told all the risks associated with each option.

The difficult question becomes how detailed to make the description of the risks and consequences. Some procedures are so simple

---

BOX 4–2 • INFORMED CONSENT DISCLOSURE REQUIREMENTS

- Nature and purpose of proposed treatment
- Material risks and consequences of proposed treatment
- Alternatives
- Consequences of refusal of treatment

and their risks so minor that informed consent is usually not obtained for them. For example, the risk of bruising and pain from a phlebotomy procedure (withdrawing blood from a vein) are common knowledge and usually not explained to the patient every time blood is drawn. However, more complicated procedures may carry significant risks. These risks are usually beyond the everyday knowledge of ordinary people. The physician should explain the risks of any kind of surgery because these risks are likely to be outside the knowledge of the ordinary individual. Further, the physician should disclose all risks that may be material and important to the patient's decision. **In the case of *Canterbury v. Spence* [3], the physician failed to inform the young patient's mother of the risk of paralysis associated with surgery to remove part of the patient's vertebrae. The court ruled that the physician violated his duty to disclose the significant dangers lurking in the proposed treatment when the mother consented to the surgery.**

In addition to disclosing the known risks of a proposed treatment, the physician must also explain to the patient the consequences of refusing the treatment. **In the case of *Truman v. Thomas* [4], the physician failed to inform the patient of the material risks of refusing recommended Pap smears between the years 1964 and 1969. The patient was diagnosed with cancer of the cervix in 1969 and died in 1970.** The court ruled that the physician breached his duty to the patient by failing to inform her of the potentially fatal consequences of allowing cervical cancer to develop undetected by a Pap smear. This case is a prime example of what has become known as the concept of **"informed refusal"** of treatment. The physician must disclose both the risks of the recommended treatment and the potential consequences of refusing the treatment.

The laws around the country have viewed the physician's duty to disclose material risks of a proposed treatment in two different ways: **(1) from the physician's perspective or (2) from the patient's perspective.** In most states, the physician's duty to disclose information will be judged against what other physicians would disclose in similar circumstances. Under this standard, the informed consent obligation is viewed from the perspective of the physician: What would a reasonable physician ordinarily think is important enough to warn the patient regarding his case? For example, if most physicians ordinarily tell their patients about a particular side effect of a drug, the physician would be faulted for not disclosing that side effect to his or her patient. The physician's actions are judged against the actions of his or her peers in the same specialty. Contrary to this perspective, in a growing number of states informed consent is viewed from the perspective of the patient. If a side effect would be significant to a patient, it should be disclosed to the patient. The fact that other physicians in the same specialty do not disclose a particular side effect or consequence of a drug or medical procedure does not relieve each individual physician of responsibility to communicate information that *a patient* would consider significant. Under this standard, the physician is required to disclose as much information as necessary to enable the patient to make a knowledgeable decision. This obligation is based on the fundamental right of a patient to make his or her own healthcare decisions based upon full knowledge of the facts.

EXCEPTIONS TO THE DUTY TO DISCLOSE

Before performing most invasive and diagnostic procedures, the patient should give informed consent authorizing the test or procedure. Usually this consent is obtained in writing. However, there may be circumstances where consent is not necessary. There may also be circumstances where there is not time or the opportunity to obtain informed consent. When the decision is made to forego obtaining informed consent, the healthcare provider must show why consent was not necessary or impossible to obtain from the patient or someone legally authorized to consent on behalf of the patient.

Minor Procedures

When a patient is admitted to the hospital, he/she ordinarily signs an admission form. This form usually contains language authorizing hospital personnel to provide care and treatment to the patient. This avoids the necessity of asking for consent every time a minor procedure is performed. Further, as has already been explained, minor procedures with minimal side effects do not require written informed consent. Procedures in this category include activities such as providing general nursing care and assistance, minor procedures such as drawing blood, and simple diagnostic tests that do not involve great risk (such as a chest x-ray).

Emergencies

The most important exception to the informed consent rule relates to emergency situations. In the case of a medical emergency where the patient is unable to communicate with caregivers, life-saving treatment may ordinarily be given without the patient's consent. The law implies consent in most emergency circumstances on the theory that if the patient were able or if a qualified legal representative were present, the consent would be given. If the patient could suffer significant harm if treatment is delayed while family is located, the physician may go forward with treatment. This exception may apply, for example, to the unconscious automobile accident victim who requires emergency surgery. However, this exception *will not apply* if evidence exists to indicate that the patient (or the patient's legal representative) would refuse the treatment.

If the patient is coherent enough to converse (such as through gestures or conversation) or if the patient's family is available, then the physician should not rely on the emergency treatment exception. Furthermore, if there is evidence that the patient would not wish the particular treatment (such as a living will expressing a desire to forego cardiopulmonary resuscitation (CPR)), then the emergency exception likely will not apply. In these situations, hospital administration should be involved to assist in resolving the problem.

Some states provide immunity to a physician who fails to obtain the patient's consent to treatment under certain emergency circumstances. For example, the California Business and Professions Code section 2397 provides that a physician is not liable for civil damages for injury or death caused in an emergency situation occurring in a physician's office or in a hospital on account of failure to obtain informed consent under any of the following conditions:

1. The patient is unconscious.

2. The physician reasonably believes that the procedure should be undertaken immediately.

3. There was insufficient time to fully inform the patient or to obtain consent from a person authorized to act on behalf of the patient.

In the case of an emergency, the physician does not sign the consent form on behalf of the patient. Rather, the patient's consent is implied by law from the existence of the emergency.

Therapeutic Exception

A controversial exception to the obligation to disclose all the risks of a proposed treatment may exist where the physician believes that informing the patient of such risks poses such a threat of harm to the patient that disclosure would be unwise or dangerous. This may occur in situations where the physician fears that the patient will become so ill or emotionally distraught upon learning of the risks that disclosure of the information would be harmful or would interfere with the patient's ability to make a rational decision. The important question for the physician in this circumstance is whether the physician is making a sound medical judgment that the disclosure would pose a risk to the patient's well-being or would interfere with the patient's ability to make a rational decision. This exception flies in the face of the fundamental principle of self-determination and has never been fully endorsed by the courts.

Waiver

Occasionally, patients may prefer to forego a discussion of the risks of a proposed treatment. Rather, these patients want to simply trust their doctors to do the best for them. In such a circumstance, the patients are making a conscious decision to choose ignorance rather than information. Essentially the patients are waiving their right to informed consent. When the patient clearly chooses not to participate in the consent process, many providers feel comfortable respecting this choice. Courts have agreed with the physicians' decisions in such circumstances. When a patient chooses to waive the right to hear all about the risks of a proposed treatment, the physician is well advised to document such waiver thoroughly in the medical record and to give the patient a number of opportunities to change his or her mind.

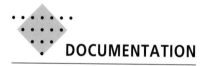

DOCUMENTATION

In all cases in which informed consent is obtained, the consent should be well documented in the patient's medical record. The person who obtained the consent, usually the physician, should prepare this documentation. In the case of emergencies, the existence of the emergency and the justification for failing to obtain consent from either the patient or a family member should also be explained.

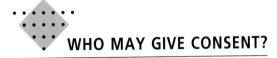

WHO MAY GIVE CONSENT?

Competent Patients

A legal and effective informed consent requires that the individual have decision-making capacity. The analysis first begins with the question of the competency of the patient. For the purpose of consenting to medical treatment, **competency may be defined as the ability to understand the nature and consequences of the procedure or treatment the patient is being asked to undergo.** The general rule is that a person is presumed to be competent unless there is valid reason to believe otherwise. If the patient is competent, then he or she may consent to any and all medical treatment. If the patient is incompetent for any reason, then consent must be obtained elsewhere.

Any number of reasons may cause incompetency. For example, individuals under the legal age of consent (18 years of age) are automatically deemed incompetent to consent to most medical treatment. (Note that this may not apply in states that permit minors the right to consent to medical treatment relating to sexually transmitted diseases and other reproductive health issues such as birth control.) Some states provide that minors who have entered into a valid marriage or who are on active duty in the armed forces of the United States of America or who have been declared emancipated pursuant to a court decision are competent to make healthcare decisions [5].

Another example of incompetency would be a patient determined by a court of law to lack the capacity to make medical decisions. These individuals usually have a "conservator of the person" appointed for them. State laws vary regarding the appointment and authority of conservators. Before relying upon the consent of a conservator, the laws in your own particular state should be explored.

Incompetency may also exist in an elderly patient with diminished mental functions, such as a person suffering from senile dementia. A formal court ruling regarding the elderly patient's capacity is not usually necessary. If the patient's treating physician or a psychiatrist is able to state that the patient lacks capacity, consent may be obtained elsewhere, such as from a "surrogate decision-maker."

However, if there is any dispute regarding the patient's capacity, recourse to the courts may be necessary.

Surrogate Decision-Maker

If an individual is thought to be incapable (incompetent) to consent to the medical treatment being offered, consent must be obtained in some other fashion. Alternative sources for consent will depend upon the reason the patient is incompetent. For example, when the patient is incompetent because of age (i.e., the patient is under 18), the healthcare provider turns to the parent or legal guardian to give consent. If a court has deemed the patient incompetent and a conservator of the person has been appointed, then one looks to the conservator to provide consent. If the patient is deemed incompetent because of mental incapacity, either temporary (such as unconsciousness due to an automobile accident) or permanent (such as senility), a hierarchy of individuals who may be capable of consenting exists. In such a circumstance, the healthcare provider should look to the following individuals to make the decision on behalf of the patient. This person is called the "surrogate decision-maker." Surrogate decision-makers include the following:

1. An adult who has been appointed by the patient to make healthcare decisions pursuant to state law (such as through a durable power of attorney for health care);

2. A conservator appointed by a court to make medical decisions; and

3. The nearest relative (spouse, parent, adult child, siblings, aunts and uncles, cousins, etc.).

Other terms commonly used include: healthcare agent, healthcare proxy, healthcare representative, and healthcare surrogate.

When none of these exist, resort to the courts for judicial permission to perform the procedure may be necessary. (It is a misconception that two physicians may agree to the need for particular treatment and consent to it on behalf of the patient when the patient is incompetent and when no surrogate decision-maker can be found. Rather, either the emergency consent rule applies or the physicians must obtain a court order authorizing the procedure. In these circumstances, legal counsel should be consulted regarding specific state laws that may apply.)

Evidence of the Patient's Desire

If the patient has made an informed decision regarding treatment prior to the onset of incapacity, that decision should be given effect even after the patient loses capacity. For example, a competent patient who instructs his or her physician to withhold CPR should have those wishes respected if the patient then loses consciousness and, thereafter, suffers a cardiac arrest.

"Living wills" or "advance healthcare directives" are documents, often handwritten, that have gained in popularity in recent years. **A living will is a declaration, signed by the patient when the patient had capacity, stating his or her wishes.** Through this document, a competent adult can provide information and direction to others regarding healthcare treatment in the event the individual is unable to make decisions for himself or herself. All states have enacted some type of law that permits competent adults to make some type of healthcare decisions in advance, which would take effect at a later date without any involvement of a court or other surrogate decision-maker. Unless the "living will" complies with the standards established by the state in which the patient is located, the living will has no legal binding effect.

Some patients may have signed a more formal document often known as an "advance healthcare directive." These directives are usually typewritten forms or documents that comply with individual state laws. As an example, California's Probate Code sets out specific requirements for what must be in an advance directive [6]. When an advance directive complies with state law, the physician may be required to follow the wishes of the patient that are expressed within that document. Further, state law may provide healthcare providers with protections from liability when the advance healthcare directive is followed. Providers should carefully check the law in their state to determine the extent to which the advance healthcare directive is binding upon them.

FOREGOING LIFE-SUSTAINING TREATMENT

When the patient is incapable of making a decision, another person is identified to make the decision on the patient's behalf (i.e., the surrogate decision-maker described above). The surrogate decision-maker must be motivated solely by an interest in the welfare of the incompetent patient. When the patient has expressed his or her desires, these statements should guide the surrogate decision-maker. When a patient has left clear evidence of his or her wishes, the surrogate decision-maker should follow these wishes. However, just as the adult competent patient has the right to refuse or decide not to receive treatment, either because it involves great pain or discomfort or is particularly intrusive or because the patient feels the time has come for treatment to stop altogether, the surrogate decision-maker has similar rights.

Despite the considerable publicity that has surrounded "right to die" issues in recent years, most patients do not leave clear evidence of their wishes. The patient may never have thought about the question or may not have been comfortable discussing his or her feelings with family members. Most courts permit other individuals to consent on the patient's behalf in these circumstances as described above. The first and most famous case to discuss the authority of a surrogate decision-maker is the **Quinlan** decision. In that case, the Supreme Court of New Jersey authorized the father of Karen Anne Quinlan to consent to have his irreversibly comatose daughter removed from a respirator. The court permitted this even though the treating physician testified that the patient would die without the respirator and that it was not the custom or practice to remove such patients under those circumstances. Given her poor prognosis, the court found no state interest that could override the patient's right to refuse treatment, which was being exercised on her behalf by her father. Other courts have since followed the New Jersey ruling and have permitted discontinuance of life support systems for irreversibly comatose patients. (In re: *Quinlan,* 355 A.2d 647 (1976).)

When an incompetent patient is severely debilitated, but not terminally ill or comatose, courts have been more reluctant to withhold medical care at the direction of the family. A significant case in this area of law is **Cruzan v. Harmon** [7]. On the night of January 11, 1983, Nancy Cruzan lost control of her car as she was driving down a road in Jasper County, Missouri. The car overturned, and Nancy was found lying face down in a ditch without detectable heartbeat or respiration. Paramedics were able to restore her breathing and heart rate at the accident site, and she was transported to a hospital unconscious. She remained in a coma for approximately three weeks and then progressed to an unconscious state in which she was able to take some nutrition by mouth. In order to ease feeding and further the recovery, surgeons implanted a feeding tube directly into her stomach. After it became apparent that Nancy had virtually no chance of regaining her mental faculties, her parents asked the hospital to stop the artificial feedings. The hospital refused to honor this request without court approval. The case made its way through the court system from the trial court level to the Missouri Supreme Court, then on to the U.S. Supreme Court. The Missouri Supreme Court ruled that in the absence of clear and convincing evidence of Nancy's wishes, the state's interest in preserving life outweighed her parents' right to refuse the life-saving treatment. For that reason, the Missouri Supreme Court refused to permit the removal of the feeding tube. The U.S. Supreme Court, in reviewing the Missouri Supreme Court's decision, supported the analysis of the Missouri court. The U.S. Supreme Court concluded that although the right to refuse treatment is supported by the United States Constitution, it is not absolute. States may set reasonable limits on the exercise of personal freedoms.

Some states, such as California, permit surrogate decision-makers broad authority to refuse or withdraw life-sustaining measures, including intravenous drips, ventilators, antibiotics, and similar treatments. However, in all circumstances, the comfort of the patient should be considered. Comfort measures, such as pain medications, may not be withheld from a dying patient.

SPECIAL CIRCUMSTANCES

Federal law specifically addresses the use of restraints in nursing home settings. In a nursing home, a special consent is required prior to the use of most types of restraints. Additionally, the Joint Commission on Accreditation of Healthcare Organizations, which accredits many hospitals and other healthcare entities, has very specific requirements regarding the application of, and consent to, restraints (see Box 4–3).

BOX 4–3 • SPECIAL CIRCUMSTANCES RELATING TO CONSENT

- Restraints
- Reproductive rights
- Mental health treatment
- Research studies
- Law enforcement

Many states have laws that permit minors, whether emancipated or not, to consent to treatment for sexually transmitted diseases. Additionally, many states give minors the authority to consent to birth control and other matters relating to pregnancy. A minor's ability to consent will vary from state to state. Some states require parental notification, such as in the case of abortion.

Patients admitted to mental health facilities have special rights regarding consent. A patient may not ordinarily be held and treated against his or her will unless careful attention is paid to complying with state and federal laws regarding involuntary commitment. It is a generally accepted principle of mental health law that even an involuntarily committed patient (that is, generally, one who has been deemed to present a clear and present danger to oneself or another) retains the limited ability to refuse certain types of medical care, such as electroconvulsive therapy ("shock treatment") and psychosurgeries such as lobotomies. State law will determine the extent of these rights.

Federal law prohibits the performance of any sort of experimental treatment for purposes of research without the express written consent of the patient or the patient's surrogate decision-maker. Further, the consent form that is used in such circumstances must comply with all of the disclosure requirements set forth in federal law. These disclosure requirements are extensive, which accounts for the lengthy and detailed consent forms used in research studies.

Not uncommonly, police officers bring a prisoner or suspect to a healthcare facility requesting that a particular medical procedure be performed on the individual. For example, a request may be made to withdraw blood for drug tests or pump the patient's stomach for collection of evidence in a drug search. Such invasive procedures may violate the patient's Fifth Amendment right against self-incrimination and the Sixth Amendment rights against unreasonable searches and seizures by law enforcement. Furthermore, if the patient objects, physical force or restraints may be necessary to enable the procedure to be performed. This may result in injury to the patient. Prior to using such force or restraint or going against the patient's wishes, the healthcare provider should check hospital or laboratory policy to determine how best to proceed.

How Consent Should Be Obtained

The obligation to provide the information necessary for the patient to give an informed consent is the responsibility of the patient's physician. Other healthcare employees involved in the consent process should merely serve as witnesses to the patient's signing of the consent form.

If the patient does not speak English, every effort must be made to provide an interpreter, either in person or by telephone. (The patient will be unable to give informed consent if he or she does not understand what is being said.) The institution in which the patient is receiving treatment should have a policy to address use of, and access to, interpreters.

When the individual giving consent is unable to sign the consent form (for example, if a spouse is providing consent over the telephone), the conversation with the surrogate decision-maker should be well documented in the patient's medical record. Some facilities require that two witnesses hear the telephone consent and that documentation describing the discussion with the decision be made a part of the chart. An explanation should be given as to why the patient or surrogate decision-maker is unable to sign the consent form. Furthermore, it is a wise practice to document all stages of the informed consent process in the medical record. Documentation of a patient's informed consent is essential for the protection of the healthcare provider and the institution.

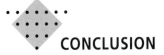

CONCLUSION

Let us revisit the case scenario in light of the information provided in this chapter. We know that, ordinarily, an adult patient is presumed competent unless we have reason to believe otherwise. We also know to look for a formal document, such as a durable power of attorney for health care or a conservatorship of the person, which may give another person the authority to make medical decisions when the patient is incompetent. We have learned that if such a document does not exist, a family member can make decisions on behalf of an incompetent patient. We also know that obtaining informed consent is the physician's responsibility and that others, such as the radiology technician, can act as a witness to the signing of the consent form.

Let us apply these lessons to the facts of the opening scenario. We see that Mrs. Richards has advanced Alzheimer's disease, which raises doubts as to whether she has the capacity to consent to the colonoscopy. The physician should evaluate the patient's ability to understand the risks and benefits of the procedure. If she cannot understand them, the physician would conclude that the patient does not have the capacity to consent. The husband should then be asked about the existence of a durable power of attorney for health care or a court-appointed conservatorship of the person. If none of these exists, the husband may be asked to sign the consent form.

When Mr. Richards began asking Susan questions about the procedure, Susan recognized that Mr. Richards did not appear to have a good understanding of the risks and benefits. Perhaps he never had the chance to speak to a physician about it, or perhaps he didn't understand the explanation given to him by the doctor. At this point, Susan should not attempt to explain the medical aspects of the procedure. Instead, she should tell Mr. Richards that it would be better if a doctor answered his questions. Susan should then find the radiologist and request that he speak directly to Mr. Richards to answer his questions. After the radiologist speaks to him, Susan may then observe Mr. Richards sign the consent form and then sign her own name as the witness.

As we can see from this scenario, knowledge of the principles of informed consent is essential to achieving the goal of providing patients with high-quality medical care. Patients deserve to have their questions answered before submitting to any medical procedure. Patients also deserve to be given enough information to make an informed decision about whether to agree to the procedure. Even though the healthcare worker may not agree with the choices made by the patient, the law requires that these choices be respected. Failure to meet informed consent obligations may result in significant liability to the healthcare provider and the employer.

PERTINENT POINTS

1. The competent adult patient has the right to accept or refuse medical procedures recommended to him or her by the physician. This right may be restricted only in limited circumstances.
2. The duty to obtain the patient's informed consent rests with the individual performing the procedure such as the physician, nurse practitioner or physician's assistant.
3. When the patient lacks capacity to consent to medical treatment, consent ordinarily may be obtained from a surrogate decision-maker. If "living will" or "natural death" legislation has been enacted in your state, then you should ask the patient

or family members whether the patient has signed a document addressing the patient's wishes regarding medical treatment.

4. In 1914, Judge Cardozo made the famous statement, "Every human being of adult years and sound mind has the right to determine what shall be done with his body."

5. A battery occurs whenever a person intentionally touches another without permission.

6. The informed consent disclosure requirements include the following:
   a. Name and proposed treatment
   b. Material risks and consequences
   c. Alternatives
   d. Consequences of refusal of treatment.

7. Exceptions to informed consent include emergencies and minor procedures.

8. A living will is a document signed by the competent patient that expresses the person's future healthcare wishes to be carried out when he or she can no longer make such decisions.

9. A medical durable power of attorney or healthcare proxy allows a patient to choose someone to make medical decisions on his or her behalf when the patient is unable to do so.

10. The physician performing the surgery or procedure should obtain informed consent from the patient.

STUDY QUESTIONS

1. Define battery and give an example.

2. Discuss the foundation for the informed consent doctrine.

3. Outline the informed consent requirements. Obtain a facility's consent form and discuss the various requirements.

4. What is the responsibility of the allied health professional with regard to informed consent forms and the process of obtaining informed consent?

5. Discuss the term "implied consent" and give an example.

6. Define the terms competency and incompetency. Discuss the general rule related to competency.

7. What is a surrogate decision-maker? Who can be a surrogate decision-maker?

8. Discuss two important legal cases relating to life-sustaining treatment and their impact on the healthcare arena. Present these cases to the class.

9. What is an advance directive? Obtain a copy of a living will and medical durable power of attorney or healthcare proxy used in a local healthcare facility and present them to the class.

10. Define the special circumstances related to consent and how they affect patient care.

REFERENCES

1. Schloendorff v. Society of New York Hospital, 211 N.Y. 125, 105 N.E. 92 (1914).
2. Cobbs v. Grant, 8 Cal.3d 229, 502 P.2d 1 (1972).
3. Canterbury v. Spence, 464 F.2d 772 (1972).
4. Truman v. Thomas, 27 Cal.3d 285 (1980).
5. California Family Code § 7122 ct seq.
6. California Probate Code §§ 4600-4805.
7. Cruzan v. Harmon, 76 S.W.2d 408 (Mo. 1988), affirmed, Cruzan v. Director, Missouri Department of Health, 110 S.Ct. 2841 (1990).

5

Documentation
and the Allied
Health Professional

PATRICIA IYER, RN, MSN

▶ Key Chapter Concepts

Medical Records
Plan of Care—Nursing Care Plan
Kardex
Progress Notes
SOAP/SOAPIE
Integrated Progress Notes
PIE Charting
Focus Charting
Flow Sheets
Graphic Sheet
Intake and Output Sheet

▶ Objectives

At the conclusion of this chapter, the reader should have a better understanding of:

1. The purposes of the medical record.

2. The major uses of the medical record.

3. The commonly used documentation forms, including a nursing care plan and kardex.

4. The components of SOAP charting.

5. The common guidelines for charting.

6. The implications of releasing confidential information about the patient.

7. The advantages and disadvantages of electronic charting.

WHY DO WE HAVE MEDICAL RECORDS?

The medical record of a patient contains a large amount of personal and medical information. The information is collected in a medical record in order to do the following:

- Help the doctors reach a diagnosis of the patient's medical condition
- Allow the nurses, therapists, and other healthcare providers to develop a list of the patient's problems
- Provide a place to record observations about the patient
- Record information about the treatments and care that are provided to the patient
- Record responses or reactions of the patient to care.

Medical records are usually created wherever a patient receives care from a healthcare professional. These locations include hospitals, homes, nursing homes, doctors' offices, outpatient clinics, urgent care centers, therapy centers (such as physical, developmental, and occupational therapy), and crisis intervention centers. The principles of recording information in a chart are similar in all of these locations.

The medical record's primary purpose is to provide a format for healthcare providers to communicate with each other concerning the patient. These individuals may include dental hygienists, radiology technologists, ultrasound technicians, nurses, doctors, dietitians, therapists, aides, social workers, and assistants. The chart allows healthcare providers who are seeing the patient at different times to learn what others have done for the patient. For example, the nurse's notes, nursing assistant's recordings, and flow sheets give the physician information about the patient's status that will affect the orders that the physician writes. The entries of a physical therapist who visits a patient at home can be used by the home health aide to reinforce the exercises that have been taught to the patient.

▶ Case Scenario

A Florida woman died in a nursing home after having been a patient for 5 years. She was 94 years at the time of admission. During her stay, she was totally dependent on skilled nursing and catheter care, but the level of care was apparently very poor. Recordkeeping was severely deficient, sometimes with gaps of weeks between the required daily nursing notes. Existing notes were often internally conflicting or in conflict with other pieces of the decedent's chart recorded on the same day by other caretakers. The woman suffered a broken ankle, broken hip, torn rotator cuff, numerous stage IV bedsores (the most serious type), and severe contractures while in the home. She died of congestive heart failure, with sepsis (blood infection) listed as a secondary cause of death. The parties settled for $800,000 two days before trial [1]. Frequency of charting was an issue in this case, which we will discuss in more detail later in the chapter.

PURPOSES OF DOCUMENTATION

The information recorded in the medical record is used to do the following:

1. Identify the patient's problems and strengths;
2. Plan care for the patient;
3. Record care that is given to the patient; and
4. Fulfill legal obligations to record pertinent information about the patient.

Patient Problem Identification

The chart consists of information about the patient's problems, which may include physical and emotional changes that affect health status. Strengths may be defined as the areas of health or the patient's abilities to care for self. For example, a patient in a nursing home may be able to wash her face and hands but needs assistance washing her back and legs. The information recorded by the nursing assistants enables others to identify the patient's abilities.

Plan Patient Care

Once the patient's problems and strengths are identified, the staff involved in the patient's care are then able to plan the care. The plan of care can be documented in several different formats. A commonly used format is a nursing care plan and critical pathway, which are described in more detail below.

Record of Care Provided

The medical record provides a format for recording care that is provided to the patient (Box 5–1). The dental hygienist records the care associated with cleaning the teeth. The home health aide documents the assistance that is provided for dressing and grooming. The medical assistant documents the patient's initial complaints when arriving at the doctor's or nurse practitioner's office. The healthcare providers use the medical record to prove that care is given which is important for reimbursement purposes and to show that the standard of care is being followed.

BOX 5–1 • COMPONENTS OF THE MEDICAL RECORD

- Plan of care
- Kardex
- Progress notes
- Flow sheets
- Graphic records

Legal Document

The medical record (chart) is a legal document and is used to determine if the healthcare providers carried out their obligations to the patient and followed policies, procedures, guidelines, and standards. It must not be thrown out, altered, or destroyed. The actual pieces of paper belong to the healthcare facility that provide the care to the patient. The patient owns the information that is recorded in the chart.

If the patient wants to read his or her record, tell the nurse, who may want to discuss this with the physician prior to showing the patient the records. Also, check to see if your hospital has a policy and procedure on allowing patients to see their charts while in the hospital. After the patient has been discharged from the facility, the patient may obtain a copy of the medical record by requesting a copy. The facility may charge a fee for duplication.

COMPONENTS OF THE MEDICAL RECORD

Plan of Care

When the patient is admitted to the facility, an initial assessment is performed. The data collected is used to identify the patient's problems and to plan the care. The plan of care may be recorded in a hospital or nursing home in the form of a nursing care plan (see Case Example 5–1). The care plan usually defines the following:

1. The patient's problems;
2. The outcomes or goals that are to be achieved; and
3. The interventions or steps to be carried out to achieve the outcomes.

Kardex

The care plan may be combined on the same piece of paper with a kardex. **The kardex is an abbreviated listing of the care**

▶ Case Example 5–1

When Mary Quigley is admitted to the nursing home, she is unsteady on her feet and at risk for falling. The nursing care plan identified for her is as follows:

Problem: High risk for falls.

Outcome: Will not fall during her stay at the facility.

Interventions:

1. Determine the reason for wanting to wander or get out of bed, such as need to use bathroom, pain, high energy level.

2. Identify the patient as fall prone by labeling the bed, the wristband, and the medical record.

3. Place recognizable symbols on the patient's door to direct the patient back to his or her own room.

4. Use bed exit alarms.

5. Place the mattress on floor.

6. Keep the call bell accessible.

The nursing care plan identifies the high-priority problems that are pertinent to the patient's condition. The nursing care plan is changed over time as the patient's needs change. After the care plan is established by the registered nurse, the licensed practical nurse may add additional information.

elements specific to the patient. The kardex commonly defines the following:

1. The type of diet;
2. The patient's activity level;
3. The amount of assistance the patient needs for bathing; and
4. The treatments that are to be performed.

Dugan, White, and Cusick [2] reported on the use of a kardex that is used by nursing assistants to identify the following:

1. The special equipment that is being used by the resident;
2. The need for a wheelchair;

3. The application schedule for splints, cones, or other rehabilitation devices;

4. Other assistive devices needed by the resident; and

5. The level of assistance the resident needs for activities of daily living.

The kardex provides a level of consistency in assignments in facilities and reduces potential errors that may be made by floating nursing assistants. The kardex is changed as the needs of the patient change.

Progress Notes

The format and design of progress notes have gone through enormous changes in the last decade. For many years, entries into medical records were written in a **narrative format**. In other words, entries were written as paragraphs with no particular organization, other than by date of entry. As health care became more complex and the need to transmit more and more information occurred, the narrative note came under attack. The criticisms of the narrative note have focused primarily on its unstructured format. It can be very difficult to locate information about a specific subject in a long narrative note. The documentation of narrative notes is very time consuming.

SOAP Format

In the 1960s, a physician by the name of Lawrence Weed created a system of organizing entries in outpatient charts. He developed the SOAP format. This system consists of a problem list and progress notes. The problem list is an ongoing listing of the patient's current and resolved problems. The progress note is broken down into four components:

S: Subjective (what the patient says)

O: Objective (what the healthcare provider observes)

A: Assessment (the conclusion of the healthcare provider about the label for the problem)

P: Plan (what will be done about the problem).

A nurse working in a facility that uses SOAP charting may make the following entry:

S: "I have pain in my abdomen."

O: Rubbing abdomen, grimacing

A: Abdominal pain

P: Give pain medication.

The SOAP system usually includes the concept of integrated progress notes. These are notes that are written on by several types of healthcare providers, such as nurses, doctors, physical therapists, dietitians, and others.

In the early 1980s, the limitations of the SOAP system became apparent as the components of the SOAP note were studied. The basic SOAP note does not include a way to document the interventions that are carried out to address the problem, nor does it include a framework for documenting the patient's response. Therefore the SOAP system has been modified to include the following:

I: Intervention (what was done about the problem)

E: Evaluation (the patient's reaction).

The full SOAPIE note may look like this:

S: "I have pain in my abdomen."

O: Rubbing abdomen, grimacing

A: Abdominal pain

P: Give pain medication

I: Demerol 75 mg IM given

E: States she felt better an hour after receiving injection.

While the new SOAPIE note provides a full framework for documenting information about the patient, the sheer length of the note makes it cumbersome to use.

PIE Charting

As the limitations of SOAPIE became clear and the time associated with writing either lengthy narrative notes or detailed SOAPIE notes became apparent, different charting systems emerged. Two of them, **PIE and focus charting,** are in common use.

PIE charting structures the progress note into P for problem, I for intervention, and E for evaluation. For example:

P: Abdominal pain

I: Demerol 75 mg IM given

E: Obtained relief within an hour.

Focus Charting

Focus charting uses a format of having a column for the focus or problem. The note is then organized into D for data, A for action, and R for response. For example:

Focus: Abdominal pain

D: Stating she has pain, clutching abdomen, grimacing

A: Demerol 75 mg IM given

R: States she received relief from pain within an hour.

Flow Sheets

As changes were made in the format of the progress note, increasing numbers of flow sheets were developed and put into use in a variety of facilities. **A flow sheet is basically a table that consists of information in columns.** A common format is to have the time of day running across the top of the page and the data elements or activities running down the length of a page.

Flow sheets on nursing units in hospitals, nursing homes, or home care address many different types of activities and needs. Commonly used flow sheets in hospitals include patient care flow sheets, care provided to a patient in restraints, neurological assessment, and vital signs. In long-term care, flow sheets typically include patient care, vital signs, and weight.

Patient care flow sheets are frequently written on by nursing assistants in hospitals and nursing homes and by home health aides. The purpose of the flow sheet is to provide a place in the chart to document the routine aspects of care, including the type of bath that is given, the patient's activity (bed rest, out of bed, bathroom

Table 5-1 Example of a Graphic Sheet

Date	Temperature	Pulse	Respirations	Blood Pressure
12/3	98.7	84	20	120/86
12/10	99.0	88	22	130/90

privileges), and the consumption of food at each meal (type of diet and percentage of food eaten).

Brief entries are written in each column. The form may include codes for entries using brief words or letters such as "C" for complete bath. Conversely, the people entering information onto the form may be recording only their initials, depending on how the form is designed. There is usually a place at the bottom of the form for providers to sign to indicate their initials and full name.

Graphic Records

A form commonly written on by nursing assistants is the **graphic sheet**. In most acute care facilities, the graphic sheet is designed so that several days' worth of data are on one form. The chart is set up so that the time (dates and hours of entries) is across the top of the page, and the vital sign values are in the left column. The form includes an area to document temperature, pulse, respiration, and blood pressure (Table 5–1). In long-term care and home care, the vital signs are taken less often. In these settings, the vital signs are usually not graphed, but are written out in longhand.

INTAKE AND OUTPUT

Forms to keep track of intake and output are commonly used in hospitals. They commonly include an area for the nurse to record the intake from intravenous fluid solutions and intravenous medications, such as antibiotics that are diluted in minibags. The nursing assistant may be involved in documenting the amount of fluids that the patient drank or the drainage from tubes. It is important that this information is as accurate as possible. A discrepancy between the patient's intake and output may result in the administration of medications or fluids to try to reestablish a balance.

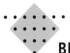

BEDSIDE DOCUMENTATION FORMS

Many acute and long-term care facilities place frequently used documentation forms at the bedside. The information may be placed on a clipboard at the end of the bed, in a box on the wall or in the hallway. The forms that are commonly found at the bedside are the graphic record and the intake and output form.

The benefits are clear-cut when considering the need for accurate, accessible information. The information that is recorded at the bedside tends to be accurate because there is no need to transcribe information from a piece of paper to a permanent record. For example, when vital signs are taken, the information is written directly on the permanent graphic record.

In older and less efficient systems, the vital signs are written on a piece of paper and put in the pocket of the nursing assistant. The information is then written on a separate sheet, which is then used by a unit clerk to record the values in the medical record.

GUIDELINES FOR CHARTING

A few good common sense rules govern the entry of information onto the medical record. The following section will define principles for charting that are common to the use of the medical record in a variety of settings and by a variety of healthcare providers.

Chart the Care You Give

In each type of patient care area, there are different rules about the frequency of charting and the types of information that should be recorded in the medical record. While charting every shift is the standard in hospitals, charting certain information every day or every week may be acceptable in long-term care. Although nurses notes are not commonly written every day in long-term care, the daily patient care flow sheet is often used daily by the nursing assistants.

In the case scenario at the beginning of this chapter, the defense of the nursing home was complicated by the absence of the required documentation. The large verdict for a patient who was 90 years of age may have been the result of the inability to point to the medical record to assert that the patient had received appropriate care.

Do Not Falsify Records

The medical record should be an accurate document that faithfully records the care that is provided. Falsifying the medical record can result in serious consequences to the patient and, for the healthcare providers, in a lawsuit, as Case Example 5–2 illustrates.

Use Ink

Since the chart is a legal document, entries must be permanent. Pencil entries are not acceptable.

▶ Case Example 5–2

The patient was admitted to the defendant hospital's Behavior Science Unit in March 1991, one day after slitting his wrist in an attempted suicide. The patient continued having suicidal thoughts while in the defendant hospital. Four days after admission, the patient took a plastic garbage can liner, which the hospital provided, and suffocated himself. The hospital's employees performed as many as 12 bed checks while the patient lay dead in his bed. The patient's death was only discovered when the hospital's staff attempted to awaken him the following morning. The Pennsylvania jury found that the hospital and the defendant physician, who treated the patient a decade earlier for depression, were grossly negligent in treating the decedent. The plaintiff received $800,000 in compensatory damages from both defendants and $800,000 in punitive damages against the hospital [3]. (Punitive damages are designed to punish the healthcare provider for conduct that is considered to be grossly negligent. Insurance policies usually do not provide coverage for punitive damages; so these awards are paid out of the pocket of the defendant.)

Corrections

If the wrong information is accidentally entered, the format for correcting this mistake is to draw a line through the entry and then write the date and the person's initials above the entry.

Avoid words that indicate negligence, such as error, mistaken entry, miscalculated, intentionally, or by accident.

Markers and Correction Fluid

The original entry should still be readable. The use of heavy black marker or correction fluid is not an acceptable method of changing the original entry. These correction methods present the appearance of an attempt to cover up or hide an error that affected the patient.

Initial or Sign the Entry

The entry should be signed by the person who put the information into the medical record. The signing of the entry provides a method of demonstrating accountability for the data and allows someone else to go back to that person to clarify the data.

Record Information With Care

The medical record acts to protect the healthcare providers when a patient has a bad outcome from care. The legal system includes the premise that the patient should make reasonable efforts to cooperate with healthcare providers and follow instructions for self care. It is important to document when the patient refuses care.

In dentists' and physicians' offices and other clinics, it is common practice to record missed appointments on a patient's chart. In Case Examples 5–3 and 5–4, the patient's failure to keep appointments and follow instructions was a factor in the successful defense of the lawsuit. Careful recording of missed appointments is essential. This is commonly written as "no show," "DNKA" (did not keep appointment), or "DNS" (did not show). Attempts to reach the patient to reschedule care, including the use of letters, post cards, or phone calls, should be documented in the medical record.

▶ Case Example 5–3

A 60-year-old Georgia truck driver had a wisdom tooth extracted by the defendant dentist. Several weeks later, another dentist diagnosed osteomyelitis (bone infection) and pathological fracture (fracture from a weakened bone) of the patient's lower jaw secondary to a postoperative infection. Surgery had to be performed to remove decayed tissue and bone and to wire the jaw. Other treatment required included intravenous antibiotics, hyperbaric oxygen treatments, and bone grafting to his jaw.

The plaintiff claimed that the extraction was unnecessary, that the defendant failed to give him appropriate postextraction instructions, and that the defendant failed to diagnose the infection during postoperative visits. The defendant contended that the extraction was necessary, that the plaintiff did not take the antibiotics as instructed, and that he did not keep all follow-up appointments. The verdict was for the defense [4]. In this case, the specific recording of missed appointments by the office staff of the dentist was a key factor in defending the dentist.

Record Unusual Incidents or Events

Unusual events are considered incidents. Descriptions of incidents are critical to document the unusual circumstances in which patients may or may not get hurt. The description of the incident is often used

▶ Case Example 5–4

A woman in her early thirties alleged that her dentist was negligent in failing to diagnose and treat periodontal disease and in failing to perform pocket depth probing or take x-rays. The defendant contended that the plaintiff declined x-rays due to the cost and that she did refer the plaintiff to a periodontist. The dentist added to her defense by maintaining that the plaintiff was contributorily negligent in missing dental appointments and that any delay in diagnosis did not affect outcome. The jury returned a defense verdict [5].

► Case Example 5–5

A 60-year-old retired woman underwent a stress echocardiogram, which included a treadmill test. A week after the treadmill test, which was done in the cardiologist's office, the woman's husband called the doctor to report that she had seriously injured her back by falling off the treadmill during the test. Neither the cardiologist nor the two technicians present in the room during the test remembered a fall or any other unusual incident occurring at the time. The plaintiff claimed that the technician had negligently instructed her to get off the treadmill while the belt was moving backward, causing her to fall and suffer a herniated disk. The defendants contended that the plaintiff injured her back sometime after the test and denied that the incident reported by the plaintiff ever happened. The verdict was for the defense [6].

The defense of the cardiologist and the technicians was based on the premise that the lack of documentation about the alleged fall indicated that it did not occur. An injury of this nature would have been recorded in the cardiologist's office notes. Additional statements by the technicians would have also been appropriate.

at the time of a lawsuit to determine if the actions of the healthcare providers are appropriate. The absence of a description of an incident may also be used to assert that a particular event did not occur (see Case Examples 5–5 and 5–6).

INCIDENT, VARIANCE OR OCCURRENCE REPORT

Documentation of incidents typically contain an objective description of the events. The report should be devoid of blame and accusations. For example, the report should not contain statements such as **"this injury occurred because we did not have enough staff to care for the patients."** The incident should be described as quickly as possible after the event so that the information is accurate. Serious incidents involving patient injury should be reported up the

▶ Case Example 5–6

In another case, the jury in a claim involving a radiology technician returned a defense verdict. The plaintiff was a man in his late
sixties who had a stroke affecting his left side. He claimed that
the day after his admission, a radiology technician came in to take
him to the radiology department for a test. The plaintiff claimed
that the technician reached over and grabbed his flaccid left arm
to get him onto the stretcher, resulting in a torn rotator cuff of
the left shoulder. The plaintiff's family, who were in the room at
the time, claimed that they complained to the attending nurse,
head nurse, and head physician, none of whom had any recollec-
tion of the complaint. There was no documentation of a complaint. The defendant denied the incident happened. The
defendant also disputed that the event occurred because the
rotator cuff tear was not diagnosed until 1 year later [7].

chain of command. Take care in filing results of diagnostic studies. It
is imperative that the results of diagnostic tests are promptly con-
veyed to the healthcare providers. Delayed reporting of critical
results can have a profound impact on the health of a patient (see
Case Example 5–7).

The accurate filing of reports is an essential responsibility of all
staff who handle medical records. Attention to detail, ensuring that

▶ Case Example 5–7

A Texas jury awarded $67.5 million to a child who lost her left leg
after her magnetic resonance imaging (MRI) result was misplaced
for more than a day. After a burro attacked her, she underwent
surgery to remove part of her intestine. A blood clot had formed
on her aorta, cutting off circulation to her leg. The results of the
MRI test were lost for more than a day. The plaintiffs argued that
the clot could have been detected and the leg saved had the
results been reported more timely [9].

▶ Case Example 5–8

In a Pennsylvania case, a 48-year-old woman underwent a mammogram in her gynecologist's office under the direction of Spectrascan employees. A Spectrascan employee misdirected the mammogram report to a pile for routine screening tests, rather than the pile for diagnostic tests. The plaintiff claimed that her breast cancer was not diagnosed between February 1995 and October 1995, allowing the cancer to spread to her bones, lungs, and brain. She was not expected to survive. A $33.1 million verdict was reached, with the gynecologist and his practice being found 17% at fault and Spectrascan being found 83% at fault. The verdict included about $1.1 million in past and future medical expenses and lost wages and $27 million to the plaintiff for pain and suffering. Her husband was awarded $5 million for loss of consortium [10].

the results are not placed on the wrong person's chart, and properly handling the report are important in managing medical records (Case Example 5–8).

CONFIDENTIALITY OF THE MEDICAL RECORD

Confidentiality of information is a primary concern of the public. Release of private health information has ruined careers and resulted in public ridicule, social rejection, and economic devastation of individuals and their families. Healthcare professionals have adopted ethical codes that address their responsibility toward protecting the privacy of patients[8]. However, there are many groups of healthcare providers who do not have formally adopted codes of ethics to guide them in making decisions about revealing patient information. Facility policies and procedures on confidentiality must also be followed. **All people involved with patient specific healthcare information are bound by an ethical code which emphasizes privacy of information [8].**

ELECTRONIC CHARTING—
COMPUTERIZED DOCUMENTATION

The issue of confidentiality assumes new importance as computerization of healthcare information becomes widespread. Security strategies are commonly used to protect the information that is contained in the computer system. **Several types of systems are used to restrict access to the computer. The use of cards to activate the terminal or passwords is commonplace. Secondary confidentiality techniques involving biometrics are also being designed. Confidentiality techniques involving retinal (eye) patterns, fingerprints, and circulatory systems checks are being developed. Once the user is admitted into the system, the information that can be accessed can be clearly defined.** For example, a nursing assistant may be allowed to enter vital sign data but could enter telephone orders from a physician or read laboratory results.

Potential Legal Problems

Computerized patient records increase the potential for legal problems through the following:

1. **Accidental or intentional disclosure of private data to unauthorized individuals;**
2. **Modification or destruction of patient records;**
3. **Entering inaccurate information into the computer; and**
4. **Making clinical decisions based on the inaccurate information [11].**

Many people feel the advantages (Box 5–2) of computerizing information outweigh the disadvantages (Box 5–3) and risk to confidentiality, provided that the users carefully respect the patient's rights.

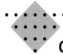

CONCLUSION

The medical record is a rich source of information about the patient. It is a convenient tool for communicating to other healthcare

BOX 5–2 • ADVANTAGES OF ELECTRONIC CHARTING

The advantages that computerizing patient information provide include the following:

1. Legible entries.
2. Instantly accessible records.
3. The potential for streamlined documentation.
4. The ability to sort and organize the data to show trends in the patient's condition.
5. Improved nursing productivity–decreases paperwork time and redundant charting.
6. Reduction in record tampering.
7. Graphical display of data so that it can be analyzed.
8. Supports the use of nursing process and individualization of patient assessment. Nursing diagnosis can be suggested by software depending on findings.
9. Automatically printed reports.
10. Documentation according to standards of care.
11. Availability of data for research projects.
12. Allows basing charges on care that is delivered.
13. Simultaneous use of patient's records.

BOX 5–3 • DISADVANTAGES OF ELECTRONIC CHARTING

1. Computer downtime–when it is not working because of sudden unexpected failure or routine servicing.
2. Size of record–may be voluminous.
3. Acceptance of computerized information when it may be incorrect.
4. Confidentiality and security issues.
5. Inadequate number of terminals.
6. Staff's difficulty in giving up worksheets.
7. Costs–hardware, software, education, and licensing fee.

providers the essential information that will help guide the care of the patient. Trends in charting include streamlined progress notes, use of computers, and increased awareness of confidentiality issues.

PERTINENT POINTS

1. The medical record contains a large amount of personal and medical information.
2. The purpose of the medical record is to provide a format for communication about the needs of the patient.
3. The information in a chart is used to identify the patient's problems and strengths, to plan and record the patient's care, and to fulfill legal obligations to record pertinent information.
4. The nursing care plan identifies the patient's problems, the goals of care, and the steps that will be taken to resolve the problems.
5. The kardex contains a quick reference to identify the needs of the patient and the treatments that have been ordered.
6. Progress notes can be structured in several different ways, including narrative, SOAP, SOAPIE, and PIE.
7. Flow sheets contain tables that are used to record information over time.
8. Forms that may be kept at the patient's bedside include graphic records, intake and output, and patient care records.
9. Guidelines for charting include the following:
   a. Chart the care you give.
   b. Do not record care that you did not provide.
   c. Use ink.
   d. Initial or sign the entry.
   e. Record information that shows the patient is not cooperative.
   f. Record information about unusual events.
10. Confidentiality is a primary concern.
11. Computerized medical records have advantages in that the information is legible, accessible, and streamlined.
12. Disadvantages of computerized medical records relate to confidentiality issues and the risk of destruction of records or entering inaccurate information into the computer.

STUDY QUESTIONS

1. Your friend says to you about a mutual acquaintance, "I think Serena had an abortion last week. Since you work as a technician in the OR, have you seen her name on the operating room schedule for an abortion?" How would you respond?

2. Your husband says to you, "Are any of the patients on your unit HIV positive and, if so, who are they?" What do you say?

3. The dietary aides say to you, "You work on Five West. I saw football star Paul Harmon's name as being on your unit. Why is he in the hospital?" How do you answer?

4. When you enter the x-ray waiting area in order to bring Mr. Watson back to his room, you find him reading his medical record. What do you do?

5. Your supervisor reviews your flow sheet after a patient has fallen out of bed and says, "I want you to chart that the side rails were up before the fall." You know that the rails were down. How do you respond?

6. You observe the unit secretary using correction fluid to change the way she transcribed a medication order. What do you do?

7. Find a healthcare provider who is using the computer for documentation. Ask that person his/her opinion about the pros and cons of the system. What are its benefits? What are its drawbacks?

8. What is the definition of a nursing diagnosis?

9. Go to your county courthouse library and ask to see a publication that reports malpractice verdicts. Make a photocopy of a case involving documentation and bring it back to the class to discuss.

10. Ask a nurse what she/he sees as the advantages and disadvantages of having flow sheets at the bedside.

REFERENCES

1. Laska, L. (Ed.) (1996, January). Elderly woman dies in nursing home. *Medical Malpractice Verdicts, Settlements and Experts,* 26–27.
2. Dugan, M., White, D., & Cusick, P. (1995, April). Care-planning in long term care. *Nursing Management, 26*(4), 48.
3. Laska, L. (Ed.) (1996, January). Pennsylvania man used garbage can bag to commit suicide. *Medical Malpractice Verdicts, Settlements and Experts,* 43.
4. Laska, L. (Ed.) (1996, February). Georgia man develops severe infection after extraction of wisdom tooth. *Medical Malpractice Verdicts, Settlements and Experts,* 8.
5. Laska, L. (Ed.) (1999, April). Failure to diagnose periodontal disease. *Medical Malpractice Verdicts, Settlements and Experts,* 7.
6. Laska, L. (Ed.) (1996, February). California woman claims she fell off treadmill during stress test and injured back. *Medical Malpractice Verdicts, Settlements and Experts,* 6.
7. Laska, L. (Ed.) (1999, April). Technician blamed for torn rotator cuff while loading patient on stretcher. *Medical Malpractice Verdicts, Settlements and Experts,* 22.
8. Milholland, K. (1994, February). Privacy and confidentiality of patient information. *Journal of Nursing Administration, 24*(2), 19–24.
9. Laska, L. (Ed.) (1999, August). Lost MRI blamed for failure to detect blood clot, resulting in child's loss of left leg and damage to nerves in right leg. *Medical Malpractice Verdicts, Settlements and Experts,* 18.
10. Laska, L. (Ed.) (1999, August). Mammogram report put in wrong pile, *Medical Malpractice Verdicts, Settlements and Experts,* 21.
11. Gobis, L. (1994, September). Computerized patient records: Start preparing now. *Journal of Nursing Administration, 24*(9), 15.

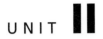

UNIT **II**

ETHICAL ISSUES

6

Legal and Ethical Issues Affecting Educators and Students

GLORIA C. RAMSEY, RN, JD

▶ Objectives

At the conclusion of this chapter, the reader will be able to:

1. Identify leading cases establishing the law for faculty and students in academic institutions.

2. Discuss how the courts determine whether an individual's constitutional rights are violated.

3. Provide key points to avoid ethical and legal problems in academic institutions.

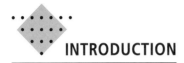

INTRODUCTION

The onslaught of court decisions for all professionals suggests that educators must know their legal rights and responsibilities. Educators must be responsible for their own competence as well as the competence of their students. Educators must assure students the necessary learning experiences to ensure that they have the skills to become competent practitioners.

In a similar vein, students demand fair treatment. Students demand an education that provides the skills expected of competent

---

▶ Case Scenario

Allen North is a dental hygienist student in his last year of college at a state institution. He met with his advisor several times and was informed, in writing and orally, that his clinical skills were not "up to par." His advisor stated on one occasion that "if he did not improve, he may be in danger of being out on probation or being dismissed from the program." Allen knows that he has been having difficulty in the clinical area. He argues that his clinical instructor, Brenda South, does not "like him." Three weeks before the end of the semester, May 30, Allen is advised by the department that he will not graduate as expected on June 15. The chair indicated that Allen's "clinical skills were unsatisfactory and his performance was below that of other students in his class." Allen is very upset and challenges the decision. What are the responsibilities of the chair? What are the responsibilities of the advisor and the clinical instructor? What are Allen's rights? Does he have any? In order to determine whether Allen has a legal right, a cause of action for the potential dismissal from the program or for the delayed graduation, we must first address the relevant law on this question. What laws might empower Allen to bring a lawsuit against the faculty challenging the faculty's evaluation and dismissal decision? What process is due to ensure that fairness will prevail?

professionals. Students demand a high-quality education in return for their high tuition costs. Accountability both to and for students has become increasingly more important. This chapter addresses rights and responsibilities of both educators and students. This chapter will carefully review the material facts set forth in leading cases that have established the law in higher education, albeit promulgated out of litigation involving medical students; however, that law is applicable to all students in academic institutions.

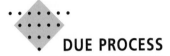

DUE PROCESS

The United States Constitution includes the **Fourteenth Amendment,** which protects certain individual rights from being restricted by state government. **The Fourteenth Amendment mandates that no state shall deprive a person of life, liberty, or property without due process of law** [1]. This provision of the amendment has been subject to great scrutiny as courts grapple with and define what due process is and, more specifically, what is life, liberty, and property. When considering the question of due process, we must first understand that due process protections are mandated only when the state is involved in restricting an individual's rights which are guaranteed by the Fourteenth Amendment. The state's involvement is often referred to as **"state action"** [2]. State action, although difficult to define what it is and what it is not, is particularly relevant when addressing whether academic institutions are public (state) or private.

Public academic institutions that are affiliated with state government are deemed state institutions and are supported by state revenues. **Private institutions** are not supported by state revenues and typically receive financial support from private funding. These distinctions are noteworthy and are material in determining liability.

The United States Constitution limits the power of the state and federal government over faculty and students in public institutions. Private academic institutions do not have the same constraints as public institutions; however, they cannot act in a manner that is **arbitrary, capricious,** or **discriminatory** when making decisions about students and faculty. Having said that, it is possible that an academic institution, even if it is private, which does receive state funds must abide by the due process requirements of the Fourteenth Amendment. Therefore, public or private institutions may be subject to due process requirements before dismissing, expelling, or suspending a student for academic misconduct.

DUE PROCESS AND THE COURTS

In 1961 in *Dixon v. Alabama State Board of Education* [3], the Court addressed the question of due process and rights of students and their relationship with the academic institution. In *Dixon,* six students at the Alabama State College for Negroes in Montgomery, Alabama, were expelled from college without notice and without a hearing for "misconduct," participating in several off-campus civil rights demonstrations. The students, after receiving a letter from the College President indicating that the Board of Education unanimously decided to expel them, filed a lawsuit requesting that the federal district court grant them a preliminary and permanent injunction restraining the Alabama State Board of Education and others from obstructing their right to attend college. The district court upheld the dismissals and denied the students' request. On appeal, the United States Court of Appeals for the Fifth Circuit reversed the district court and remanded the case back to the circuit court for further proceedings.

The appeals court, upon reviewing the trial court's decision, held that the due process protections guaranteed in the Fourteenth Amendment of the United States Constitution required a state academic institution to give notice to students concerning their possible expulsion and a hearing prior to the expulsion. The court also held that the following **standards** should be applied when providing notice and hearing:

1. The notice should be specific as to the charges and basis for the expulsion.

2. The nature of the hearing should be dependent on the circumstances of each case but should allow an opportunity for both sides to present in detail their respective positions [4].

In addition, the *Dixon* court held that the students must be given the names of witnesses against them, what each witness would be testifying to, the opportunity to present their own defenses to the charges, and, if the hearing was to be held before the State Board of Education, a written copy of its findings and decision in the case [5].

Dixon was a leading case for students in postsecondary public academic institutions when threatened with expulsion, suspension, and/or a disciplinary action. This case promulgates that "fair play, due process" mandate that notice and some opportunity for a hearing is required before a student at a **tax-supported college** is expelled for misconduct. The court further reasoned that the right to notice and a hearing is so fundamental to the conduct of our society that the waiver must be clear and explicit [6]. Disciplinary dismissals against a student are a serious matter and can have an everlasting effect on the student's reputation and standing in the community. Without an education, students may not be able to earn an adequate livelihood or complete the duties and responsibilities of good citizens [7]. Academic dismissals are considered a serious offense.

Moreover, in 1969 the United States Supreme Court in *Tinker v. Des Moines Independent Community School District* [8] recognized that school officials do not possess absolute authority over their students. Students "in" school as well as "out" of school are persons under our constitution. They are possessed of fundamental rights that the states must respect, just as the students themselves must respect their obligations to the state [9]. **In a similar vein, the United States Supreme Court in *Goss v. Lopez* [10] required that all public academic institutions provide due process protections to their students.** The *Goss* decision involved nine public high school students who filed a class action suit against the Columbus Board of Education and various administrators alleging that the students were all suspended—without a hearing—for misconduct for up to 10 days. The students alleged that the Ohio statute was unconstitutional in that it allowed a school principal to suspend a student without a hearing prior to the suspension [11]. The students alleged that the lack of a hearing was a violation of their procedural due process rights guaranteed by the Fourteenth Amendment of the United States Constitution. Accordingly, they sought to enjoin the public school officials to remove a reference to their suspension from their record [12].

The federal district court did the following:

1. **Found that the students were denied their due process rights;**

2. **Found that the Ohio statute permitting a suspension to occur without prior hearing, or within a reasonable time period after the suspensions, was unconstitutional; and**

3. **Ordered that any and all reference to the students' suspensions be removed from the school record.**

Furthermore, the court declared that there are minimal requirements that a school must undertake before a suspension is to take place. The court stated that relevant case authority would:

1. Permit immediate removal of a student whose conduct disrupts the academic atmosphere of the school;
2. Require notice of suspension proceedings to be sent to students' parents within 24 hours of the decision to conduct the proceedings;
3. Require a hearing to be held, with the student present, within 72 hours of his or her removal [13], and such a hearing should provide at a minimum
   a. production of statements in support of the charge(s) upon which the hearing is conducted
   b. statements by the student and others in explanation or mitigation of the student's conduct
   c. that the school permit an attorney to be present
   d. that the school should within 24 hours advise the student and his or her parents by letter of its decision and the reasons therefore [14].

Although the court is silent regarding the documentation of this process, it is prudent for educators to document the process to create a paper trail that refutes any disparate treatment.

The defendants appealed the district court holding to the United States Supreme Court, and on appeal, the court affirmed the lower court's holding. Accordingly, the court held that the **property right** created by Ohio in its statute for a free public education to all residents between the ages of 5 and 21 years of age and the state's requirement of compulsory attendance in school for an identified period of time, was one that could not be taken away in violation of the Fourteenth Amendment requirement of due process. The court further reasoned that because a suspension may result in a student's good name or reputation being damaged among fellow pupils and teachers, as well as interfere with later opportunities for higher education and employment, the Constitution demanded that due process protections be adhered to. The court held that some kind of notice and a hearing are necessary before a suspension takes place. This requirement is imperative if we are to protect students' due process rights and to "prove a meaningful hedge against erroneous action" [15].

The *Dixon* and *Goss* courts addressed the question of disciplinary actions in public institutions. However, an equally compelling question is what are the rights of students when an academic institution dismisses a student from the program. In 1978 the United States Supreme Court in *Board of Curators of the University of Missouri v. Horowitz* [16] dealt with this question.

In *Horowitz* [17], Charlotte Horowitz, a former medical student, was admitted with advanced standing to the University of Missouri—Kansas City (UMKC) School of Medicine in the fall of 1971. During the final year of a student's education at the medical school, the student is required to pursue in "rotational units" academic and clinical studies pertaining to various medical disciplines such as obstetrics-gynecology, pediatrics, and surgery. Each student's academic performance at the school is evaluated on a periodic basis by the **Council on Evaluation,** a body composed of both faculty and students, whose role is to recommend various actions, including probation and dismissal. The recommendations of the council are reviewed by the **Coordinating Committee,** a body composed solely of faculty members, and must ultimately be approved by the **Dean.** Students are not typically allowed to appear before either the council or the Coordinating Committee when the student's academic performance is reviewed [18].

In the spring of Horowitz's first year of study, several faculty members expressed dissatisfaction with her clinical performance during a pediatrics rotation. The faculty members noted that Horowitz's "performance" was below that of other peers in all clinical patient-oriented settings. She was also erratic in her attendance at clinical sessions and lacked a critical concern for personal hygiene. Upon the recommendation of the Council on Evaluation, Horowitz was advanced to her second and final year on a probationary basis [19].

The faculty remained dissatisfied with Horowitz's clinical performance during the following year. In fact, Horowitz's faculty advisor rated her clinical skills as "unsatisfactory." In the middle of the year, the council again reviewed Horowitz's academic progress and concluded that she should not be considered for graduation in June of that year. Furthermore, the council recommended that, absent "radical improvement," Horowitz be dropped from the school [20].

In the meantime, Horowitz was permitted to take a set of oral and practical examinations as an "appeal" of the decision not to permit her to graduate. In accordance with this "appeal," Horowitz spent a substantial portion of time with seven practicing physicians in the area who enjoyed a good reputation among their peers. The physicians were asked to recommend whether Horowitz should be allowed to graduate on schedule and, if not, whether she should be dropped immediately or allowed to remain on probation. Only two of the physicians recommended that Horowitz be able to graduate on schedule. Of the other five, two recommended that she be immediately dropped from the school. The remaining three recommended that she not be allowed to graduate in June and be continued on rotation pending further reports on her clinical progress. Upon receipt of these recommendations, the Council on Evaluation reaffirmed its prior position [21].

The council met again in mid-May to consider whether Horowitz should be allowed to remain in school beyond June of that year. Noting that the report on Horowitz's recent surgery rotation rated her performance as "low-satisfactory," the council unanimously recommended that "barring receipt of any reports that Miss Horowitz has improved radically, [she] not be allowed to re-enroll in the ... School of Medicine" [22]. The Council delayed making its recommendation official until receiving reports on other rotations. **When a report on Horowitz's emergency rotation also turned out to be negative, the council unanimously reaffirmed its recommendation that Horowitz be dropped from the school. The Coordinating Committee and the Dean approved the recommendation and notified Horowitz of their decision. Horowitz appealed the decision in writing to the University's Provost for Health Sciences. The Provost sustained the school's actions after reviewing the record compiled during the earlier proceedings. Horowitz then sued the medical school of a public university challenging her dismissal.** The United States District Court for the Western District of Missouri entered judgment for the University's Board of Curators, and the medical student appealed. The United States Court of Appeals [23] reversed and remanded and denied an **en banc** rehearing [24]. **Certiorari was granted to the United States Supreme Court to consider what procedures must be accorded to a student at a state educational institution whose dismissal may constitute a deprivation of "liberty" or "property" within the meaning of the Fourteenth Amendment. The U.S. Supreme Court held the following:**

1. **A student who was fully informed of faculty dissatisfaction with her clinical progress and the consequent threat to her graduation and continued enrollment was accorded procedural academic due process notwithstanding the lack of a formal hearing.**

2. **Academic deficiency dismissals do not necessitate a hearing before a school's decision-making body.**

3. The record revealed no showing of arbitrariness or capriciousness which would warrant remand of the case for consideration of deprivation of substantive due process.

The United States Supreme Court noted that they need not decide whether Horowitz's dismissal deprived her of a liberty interest in pursuing a medical career. They also did not have to decide whether Horowitz's dismissal infringed any other interest constitutionally protected against deprivation without procedural due process. The school fully informed respondent of the faculty's dissatisfaction with her clinical progress and the danger that this posed to timely graduation and continued enrollment. The ultimate decision to dismiss Horowitz was careful and deliberate. These procedures were sufficient under the Due Process Clause of the Fourteenth Amendment. The U.S. Supreme Court agreed with the district court that Horowitz "was afforded full procedural due process by the [school]" [25].

In *Goss v. Lopez* [26], the United States Supreme Court held that due process requires, in connection with the suspension of a student from public school for disciplinary reasons, "**that the student be given oral or written notice of the charges against him and, if he denies them, an explanation of the evidence the authorities have and an opportunity to present his side of the story**" [27]. All that *Goss* required was an informal "give-and-take" between the student and the administrative body dismissing him that would, at least, give the student "the opportunity to characterize his conduct and put it in what he deems the proper context" [28].

In *Goss,* the court felt that suspensions of students for disciplinary reasons have a sufficient resemblance to traditional judicial and administrative fact finding to call for a "hearing" before the relevant school authority.

Academic evaluations of a student, in contrast to disciplinary determinations, bear little resemblance to the judicial and administrative fact-finding proceedings to which we have traditionally attached a full-hearing requirement. In *Goss,* the school's conclusions were that the individual students had participated in demonstrations that had disrupted classes, attacked a police officer, or caused physical damage to school property. Like the decision of an individual professor as to the proper grade for a student in his course, the determination of whether to dismiss a student for academic reasons requires an expert evaluation of cumulative information and is not readily adapted to the procedural tools of judicial or administrative decision making [29].

Even assuming that the courts can review under such a standard an academic decision of a public educational institution, we agree with the district court that no showing of **arbitrariness** or **capriciousness** has been made in this case. Courts are particularly ill equipped to evaluate academic performance [30].

The court, after reviewing the evidence in some detail, concluded, "The evidence presented in this case totally failed to establish that Horowitz was expelled for any reason other than the quality of her work" [31].

ACADEMIC DUE PROCESS

Seven years later, in 1983, a second landmark decision [32] **involving academic due process and postsecondary students was made** *(Regents of University of Michigan v. Ewing)*. In the fall of 1975, Ewing entered the University of Michigan, a public university, Inteflex program, a 6-year program where students earned both a bachelor's degree and a degree in medicine. His academic performance throughout the program was complicated by a number of personal and academic problems. After 6 years of being enrolled in the Inteflex program, Ewing took part I of the National Board of Medical Examiners (NBME) examination, a required examination before students are able to go into the clinical component of the program. All medical students at the University of Michigan were required to pass the exam with a score of 345 or higher before beginning their clinical rotations. Ewing received a score of 235, the lowest score ever recorded at the University of Michigan [33].

After the examination, the Promotion and Review Board unanimously voted to drop Ewing from the program. Ewing met with the board following his dismissal and explained the several events that gave rise to his poor performance. His mother had a heart attack, he and his girlfriend of 5-1/2 years ended their relationship, and he spent considerable time writing a paper for an essay contest. Ewing reminded the board of the time and effort he had already invested in the program and his deep desire for a career in medicine. He cited the excellent clinical work that he had done [34].

Ewing filed suit in the district court when the Promotion and Review Board did not grant Ewing's request. The district court agreed that Ewing **had a property interest in his continued enrollment in the Inteflex program. The issue before the court was whether and to what extent academic decisions as to the qualifications of a** medical student are subject to substantive due process [35]. The test to determine a violation of substantive due process, which this court noted that it had outlined in an earlier decision [36], and which Ewing needed to establish, is that there was "no rational basis for the university's decision" or that the decision to dismiss him was "motivated by bad faith or ill will unrelated to academic performance" [37]. **The district court found for the university and concluded that the university did not act in violation of Ewing's due process rights.** There had been no allegations that the university's decision was based on bad faith, ill will, or other impermissible ulterior motives. The evidence demonstrated that the decision to dismiss Ewing was reached in a fair and impartial manner and only after careful and deliberate considerations [38]. "Even after a traditional substantive due process review, the court found that the evidence demonstrates no arbitrary or capricious action since the university had good reason to dismiss Ewing from the program" [39]. Moreover, the court held that Ewing did not have a **contract right** that required the university to give him a second chance to take part I of the NBME examination.

Ewing appealed the district court's ruling to the U.S. Court of Appeals for the Sixth Circuit, which agreed with the district court that Ewing had a property interest in his continued enrollment in the Inteflex program. The court held that "an implied understanding that a student shall not be arbitrarily dismissed from his university is a property interest, resting in the contractual relationship between the parties which can give rise to constitutional protections" [40]. The university argued that Ewing's dismissal was not arbitrary or capricious and cited the Medical School Bulletin that noted the Promotion and Review Board had broad discretionary power to dismiss students who did not meet academic qualifications [41]. The U.S. Court of Appeals for the Sixth Circuit reviewed the evidence and looked closely at a university document entitled "On Becoming a Doctor." The pamphlet stated that "a qualified student should be given a second chance to take the NBME" [42]. Ewing did not learn of the pamphlet's contents before taking the exam, but the court noted, "this pamphlet memorialized the consistent practice of the medical school with respect to students who initially fail that examination" [43]. **Therefore, the court held that "the university treated Ewing in an arbitrary and capricious manner by not allowing him a second opportunity to take part I of the NBME"** [44]. At trial, the testimony did not determine Ewing's status as a qualified or unqualified student. **Accordingly, the court of appeals reversed the decision of the district**

court and remanded with instructions that Ewing be allowed to retake part I of the NBME and be reinstated to the Inteflex program if he passed the exam [45].

The University of Michigan petitioned the United States Supreme Court for a writ of certiorari to "consider whether the court of appeals had misapplied the doctrine of substantive due process" [46]. The court agreed with the district court and the court of appeals that Ewing had a property interest in continued enrollment in the Inteflex program [47].

The issue before the court was "whether the record compels the conclusion that the university acted arbitrarily in dropping Ewing from the Inteflex program without permitting re-examination of part I of the NBME" [48].

The court noted that the fact that the university did not permit Ewing to retake the NBME examination was not actionable in and of itself. However, the refusal to allow Ewing to retake the examination was important to his claim that his dismissal was arbitrary and capricious [49]. The court further noted that this is not a case in which the procedures used by the university were unfair or that the regents concealed nonacademic or constitutionally impermissible reasons for expelling Ewing. The district court found that the regents acted in good faith [50]. Ewing was dismissed on the basis of his entire academic record and according to procedures outlined in the university catalog.

Here the court did not find that the university deprived Ewing of his due process rights and acted arbitrarily in dropping Ewing from the Inteflex program without permitting a re-examination. Accordingly, the U.S. Supreme Court did not agree with the reasoning of the Court of Appeals for the Sixth Circuit that Ewing's rights were violated and therefore reversed its decision.

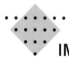

IMPLICATIONS FOR FACULTY AND STUDENTS

The *Horowitz* and *Ewing* decisions defined the rights to due process in academic matters on the public postsecondary campus. Students in cases since *Horowitz* and *Ewing* have claimed a **property right** in terms of admission to a program of study, continued enrollment, better grades, taking examinations, and receiving a degree [51]. In terms of **liberty relationships,** students have claimed a right to reputation or good name and the right to pursue a career [52].

Accordingly, in cases involving adverse academic decisions, all the procedural due process that is required is that students receive advance notice of the grading requirements and/or performance evaluations, specifically, notice of the academic rule. Academic rules include being informed in advance of grading policies for courses and course requirements for programs of study through such mediums as catalogs and syllabi, as well as being informed of performance deficiencies and negative consequences in person or in writing [53].

In the case of Allen North, the *Horowitz* and *Ewing* cases, in particular, suggest a framework to analyze whether Allen was treated fairly. We need to explore whether there was sufficient notice, whether the statement made by the advisor and chair constituted notice, and whether the decision was arbitrary and capricious or careful and deliberate. In addition to these questions, it is important that students and faculty remember these key points.

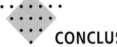

CONCLUSION

If faculty and students abide by the key points identified, both faculty and students will avoid unethical conduct and minimize the need for litigation. Courts have repeatedly held that it is not the best forum to resolve these disputes. Therefore, it is up to educators to know what law is established and what ought to be done to ensure that fairness is afforded to all.

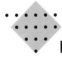

PERTINENT POINTS

1. Know your academic institution's policies on admission, dismissal, suspension, expulsion, and readmission.
2. Read your academic institution's policy statements in academic catalogs and department and/or program handbooks.
3. Follow the policy and procedures and other documents as delineated. The materials must be clear, unambiguous, and state what is intended by the academic institution.
4. Know whether the academic institution has any disclaimers in the institution's catalog or other documents thereby giving it the right to make changes including, but not limited to, changes

in the curriculum, course content, and other areas as it deems appropriate.

5. Establish an objective method to evaluate student, classroom, and clinical performance. *Horowitz* established that the court will not interfere with academic decision making because it is not equipped to evaluate an academic setting. Notwithstanding, the court will carefully review whether faculty decisions are any of the following:

   a. Arbitrary, capricious, malicious, and not in accordance with stated policies and procedures
   b. In bad faith
   c. Violative of the student's due process rights.

6. The court will override academic decisions if there is a clear departure from "accepted academic norms that demonstrate that the person responsible did not exercise professional judgment."

7. Provide students with a copy of the evaluation tool on the first day of class so that they are put on notice as to how they will be evaluated.

8. Evaluate the student throughout the clinical rotation. If the student is not meeting the clinical objectives, the student must be warned and told how to improve and what time constraints are placed in which to make those improvements. In addition, the student must be informed of what will happen if the improvements do not occur. For example, suspension, expulsion, dismissal, request for withdrawal, or receiving an "F" grade.

9. Grade students in accordance with stated policy.

10. Faculty must put in writing what is said to the student and include it in the student's permanent record.

STUDY QUESTIONS

1. What is due process?

2. Discuss the Fourteenth Amendment and how it affects the rights of students.

3. How can educators protect their university from lawsuits involving students who fail courses or clinicals?

4. What is the grievance procedure in your school?

5. Discuss when faculty decisions may be reviewed by the courts.

6. Discuss your catalog and policy and procedures on admission, suspension, dismissal, and readmission.

7. Create an objective method to evaluate student, classroom and clinical performance and present it to the class.

8. Discuss one type of evaluation tool used—the pros and cons and how it can be changed and used for other courses.

9. In your school, what actions or inactions will result in suspension, expulsion, and dismissal?

10. Select one of the cases mentioned in the readings. Determine if any newer cases have been reported on the issues tried in the case you selected.

11. Discuss one leading case that addresses a student's rights and due process.

12. Define arbitrary, capricious, and discriminatory.

13. Give examples of "property rights" that students may claim in a lawsuit.

14. Give examples of "liberty relationships" that students may claim in litigation.

15. List three key points that educators should follow when teaching students.

16. List three key points that students should know relating to admission, dismissal, suspension, expulsion, and readmission.

REFERENCES

1. U.S. Constitution, Amendment XIV, subsection 1.
2. Chandler, R., Enslen, R., and & Renstrom, P. (1993). *Constitutional law handbook* (2nd ed.) (p. 697). Rochester, N. Y.: Lawyers Cooperative.
3. Dixon v. Alabama State Board of Education, 294 F.1d 150 (5th Cir.), cert. denied, 368 U.S. 930, 82 S.Ct. 368, 7 L.Ed.2d 193 (1961).
4. Id. at 158-159.
5. Id.

6. Id. at 156.
7. Id.
8. Tinker v. Des Moines Independent Community School District, 393 U.S. 503, 509 (1969).
9. Id. at 511.
10. Goss v. Lopez, 419 U.S. 565, 95 S.Ct. 729, 42 L.Ed.2d (1975).
11. Id. at 567, 95 S.Ct. at 732.
12. Id.
13. Id. at 572.
14. 375 F.Supp. 1279, 1302. See also supra note 10 at 572.
15. Supra note 10, at 741.
16. Board of Curators of the University of Missouri v. Horowitz, 435 U.S. 78, 98 S.Ct. 948, 55 L.Ed.2d 124 (1978).
17. Id.
18. Id. at 79.
19. Id. at 81.
20. Id.
21. Id. at 82.
22. Id.
23. 538 F.2d 1371 (1976).
24. 542 F.2d 1335 (1976).
25. Regents of University of Michigan v. Ewing, 559 F.Supp. 791 (1983), 474 U.S. 214 (1985).
26. Id. at 794.
27. Id. at 796.
28. Id. at 584 .
29. Cafeteria Workers v. McElroy, 367 U.S. 886, 895, 81 S.Ct. 1743, 1748, 6 L.Ed.2d 1230 (1961).
30. Id. at 92.
31. Id. at 94.
32. Regents of University of Michigan v. Ewing, 559 F.Supp. 791 (1983), 474 U.S. 214 (1985).
33. Id. at 794.
34. Id. at 796.
35. Id. at 797.
36. 435 U.S. 78 (1978).
37. Supra note 36 at 797.
38. Id. at 799.
39. Id. at 800.
40. 742 F.2d 913, 915 (1984).
41. Id. at 915.
42. Id. at 916.
43. Id.
44. Id.
45. Id.
46. 474 U.S. 214 (1985).
47. Id. at 222-223.
48. Id.
49. Id. at 224.
50. Id. at 225.
51. Ford, D. L., & Stope, J. L. (1986). Judicial responses to adverse academic decisions affecting public postsecondary institution students since "Horowitz" and "Ewing." *Educational Law Reporter, 110, 517.*
52. Id. at 110.
53. Clements v. The County of Nassau, 835 F.2d 1000 (2nd Cir. 1987).

7

Ethical Issues in Health Occupations

BARBARA EDWARDS, RN, MTS

▶ Key Chapter Concepts

Ethics
Ethical Dilemma
Morals
Bioethics
Autonomy
Beneficence
Nonmaleficence
Professional Ethics
Justice

▶ Objectives

At the conclusion of this chapter, the reader should have a better understanding of:

1. The definition of morals.

2. The definition of a moral dilemma.

3. The definition of ethics.

4. Moral principles that healthcare practitioners try to uphold in a moral dilemma.

5. Approaches to solving an ethical problem.

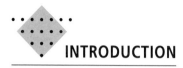

INTRODUCTION

When healthcare workers hold patients' lives in their hands, they must know the right thing to do when complications arise. Most healthcare training focuses on what steps should be taken when medical emergencies or clinically related problems (e.g., bleeding—apply pressure) arise.

In addition to clinical/medical complications, healthcare professionals must also deal with complicated ethical dilemmas. For example, suppose the person who is bleeding is HIV positive? What if the person feeling faint is not a patient? Should rescue breathing be started on someone who did not want heroic measures done to save his life? These are ethical dilemmas, and the healthcare worker entrusted with the well-being of his or her patients must know—or be able to discern—what is the right and wrong thing to do. Ethics is the way to decide what is the right thing to do in the case of a moral dilemma.

DEFINING TERMS

What makes something right, and what makes something wrong? Usually, the answer lies in the religious, cultural, and political heritage we have received. People have been arguing about what is right and what is wrong for thousands of years. And yet, despite the variety of religions and political systems in the world, there is some agreement. For example, most people believe that killing is wrong. The belief that killing is wrong is a moral belief. **Morals are ideas about right and wrong.** Killing is wrong, helping the poor is right, stealing is wrong, and easing pain is right; these are all widely shared moral ideas.

Morals should not be confused with cultural habits or customs such as wearing certain types of clothing. Morals tend to be deeply ingrained into a culture or religion and are often part of its identity.

▶ Case Example 7–1

> A dental assistant is working with a dentist in the examination of a new patient. The patient has a severely abscessed tooth and will require extensive root canal work. As the assistant prepares for the invasive procedure, the patient mentions that his lover has recently died of AIDS and that he, too, has AIDS. The assistant freezes. He is afraid of getting infected with the AIDS virus. Can he refuse to assist in this procedure?

A moral dilemma occurs when moral ideas conflict. The death penalty is an example of a moral dilemma. The morals in conflict are the ideas that killing is wrong, but punishing criminals is right. Many people have argued long and hard on both sides of the death penalty issue but have been unable to agree. The reason they do not agree is because two good moral ideas are in conflict, and it is not clear which "side" to take. In health care, many moral dilemmas exist. What should be done about the patient described in Case Example 7–1?

The moral dilemma in Case Example 7–1 is as follows: It is good to help people in need, but it is good to protect yourself from harm. The conflict exists because the patient needs help, but by helping, the healthcare professional may be putting herself in danger by coming into contact with infected blood.

Ethics is the process of deciding what is the right thing to do in a moral dilemma. Ethics is deciding right from wrong. Ethics is about making decisions. Ethics is about acting on the basis of what is right. Ethics can be defined as declarations of what is right or wrong and of what ought to be.

Ethics exists in all professional fields, e.g., business ethics, journalistic ethics, and political ethics. **Ethics that deal with patients and health care is often termed "bioethics."**

The center of health care is always the patient's need. No healthcare worker has the luxury to step back when a dilemma occurs, go home, and think about things for a while. It is also not permissible for the healthcare worker to decide that someone else with more training, knowledge, or power will figure out what to do. When the patient presents a dilemma, it is every healthcare worker's responsibility to determine what is in the patient's best interest (Case Example 7–2).

▶ Case Example 7-2

A nurse's aide in a hospital is making rounds to pick up lunch trays. An elderly patient has not eaten her food—again. The aide asks if the patient wants her lunch to be heated. The patient shakes her head no. "Please just tell them I ate everything. I don't want any more food. I just want to die." The aide leaves the room with the tray but is upset. Without food, the patient will starve to death. If she lies to the nurse at the patient's request, is she helping the patient commit suicide? Can a competent adult refuse to eat? Is the patient competent?

A SHORT HISTORY OF BIOETHICS

Medicine had little to offer patients beyond hope, kind words, and often unscientific treatments that held a high mortality rate until the discovery of germ theory and antibiotics in the late 19th and early 20th centuries. Until then, there was little ethical debate.

Active, focused bioethical debate did not begin until this century, when many major medical advances were made. Some bioethical topics have risen, fallen, and risen again. For example, in the 1920s, euthanasia societies in the United States began the push for legalized suicide. This movement fizzled with the discovery of the massive euthanasia of the Jews and others by the Nazis in World War II. However, with all the discussion in the 1970s and 1980s of the withdrawal of life support to end suffering lives, assisted suicide has risen again as an important topic of debate in the field of bioethics. Several states have proposed legislation to legalize assisted suicide, and one—Washington State—has succeeded.

Medical research is another topic of bioethical debate in this century. With the discovery that medical experiments were performed on Jews by the Nazis, there was wide agreement that medical experiments should meet certain criteria and that people must agree to serve as research subjects. And yet, in the 1960s and 1970s, it was revealed that American researchers performed harmful experiments on black men and retarded children without their consent. In response, committees called **institutional review boards (IRBs)** were established to review all research proposals and make sure that all research standards were met and that research subjects were given the opportunity to understand and consent to the research. These IRBs have been in wide use since the 1970s. In the 1990s, it was again being debated whether consent of the research subjects is always required.

The **withdrawal of life support** has been another subject of a great deal of debate in the latter half of the 20th century. With the wide use of intravenous (IV) solutions after World War II, Roman Catholics—who operate hospitals all over the United States—began to debate whether IV fluids were ethically required therapy for dying patients.

Advances in medical science in the 1960s brought open-heart surgery, the first organ transplants, the first intensive care units, kidney dialysis, and cardiopulmonary resuscitation. These advancements set the stage for bioethical debates about withdrawing some of this aggressive, highly technological medical care when it did not benefit the patient. In 1970, the **Karen Ann Quinlan** case was before the medical community. The **Harvard "brain death" criteria** were introduced, and there were fierce debates over the ethics of withdrawing life support and the very first bioethics committees evolved.

By the 1980s, the withdrawal of life support issues evolved into debates about **do not resuscitate (DNR) orders.** As in Case Example 7–2, the withdrawal of feeding was the subject of many court cases. The use of **living wills** began to block the use of aggressive medical care before it could be started. Bioethics committees spread into hospitals in every state.

In the 1990s, the debates about the withdrawal of life support shifted slightly to focus on **assisted suicide, futile medical care, durable power of attorney, and the place of economics in making decisions about expensive medical care.** Ethics committees flourished in hospitals and spread into nursing homes, hospices, and visiting nurse associations throughout the country.

Many other bioethical issues have been debated in the 20th century as well. The national debates in the 1960s over **birth control** and **abortion** spurred ethical debate among healthcare professionals. Highly technological and expensive treatment to help **childless couples** become parents began in the 1970s with the birth of the first **"test tube" baby** and has been hotly debated ever since. **AIDS** "arrived" in the early 1980s and has been the subject of debate ever since.

Continuing bioethical debate in the United States is over how to pay for health care for the millions in this country who do not have healthcare insurance. Is health care a right or a service that one should pay for? How much health care should Medicare and Medicaid recipients receive—a bare minimum or everything from antibiotics to expensive organ transplants?

As health care has become more complex, more technological, and more expensive, the bioethical dilemmas facing healthcare workers have become common. Most hospital deaths now occur to patients with DNR orders, for example. Millions of Americans are not covered by any kind of health insurance, and a significant percentage of children are not up to date on required immunizations for deadly diseases.

All of these bioethical problems are realistic, daily issues in health care today. All healthcare workers will face some bioethical dilemmas in their practice (Case Example 7–3). It is important to examine these issues thoroughly. Thinking about these difficult problems ahead of time prepares the healthcare professional to deal with them in practice so that the patient can be better served.

▶ Case Example 7–3

A nurse's aide has been employed by a family to take care of a 7-year-old girl severely brain damaged in a near-drowning accident when she was 3. During the 3 months the aide has been employed, he has gotten to know his young patient well. Although the girl cannot talk, he has learned what foods she likes and does not like, that she sleeps better if she is placed on her right side, that she cries whenever she hears loud noises, and that she likes to listen to music. One day, the aide accompanies the patient and her mother to a doctor's office—the patient needs minor surgery on her hand to remove a small cyst, and that will be done in the doctor's office. The doctor asks the aide to stay with the child to help hold her hand in place while the minor surgery is done. The aide notices that the doctor is not preparing to give the child a numbing shot on her arm where the surgery is to be done. The aide asks about this, and the doctor states, "She doesn't need anything. She's just a vegetable."

BOX 7–1 • APPROACH TO BIOETHICAL DILEMMA

1. **Identification**—Identify the problem. What morals are involved? Which morals are in conflict?

2. **Information**—Get as much information as possible about the problem.

3. **Communication**—Talk with other healthcare personnel on the case. Do they think there is a problem too? Do they agree with your understanding of the problem? Talk to your supervisor.

4. **Choice**—When all the talking is done, a choice needs to be made about what to do about the problem. A choice *must* be made. Even choosing not to decide is to decide.

APPROACHING A BIOETHICAL DILEMMA

Many bioethical problems are difficult. Usually the morals that are in conflict are good moral ideas. Usually the people involved are trying to do the right thing for the patient. But still it is not clear what is the right thing to do. How can it be sorted out? The first move is to apply the four steps in approaching a bioethical dilemma (Box 7–1). How should the nurse's aide in Case Example 7–3 begin to solve this moral dilemma? Where should any health care professional begin when faced with a bioethical problem?

STEPS IN RESOLVING AN ETHICAL DILEMMA

Identify the Dilemma or Problem

First of all, the healthcare worker should **identify** that this is a moral dilemma. Remember, morals are ideas about right and wrong. A moral dilemma occurs when two morals are in conflict. In Case

Example 7–3, the morals that are in conflict are that it is right to protect your patient and that it is also right to work with other healthcare professionals to take care of the patient. Here, the aide either needs to stay silent and allow his patient to be subjected to pain, or he needs to speak up—possibly angering the physician—in order to protect his patient. What should be done?

Obtain Information

Before anything is done, get as much **information** about the problem as possible. This is an essential step because often the drama or pressure of a difficult bioethical problem excites or intimidates people in the case. Hasty decisions may be made without all the facts. In Case Example 7–3, it would be helpful to know if this doctor has performed minor surgery on this child before. Does he know whether or not she requires local anesthesia? Does this type of surgery tend to cause pain on patients?

Communicate the Problem

It is absolutely necessary to **communicate** about the problem with the people involved in the patient's care. People involved in a patient's care include everyone from other healthcare providers— nurses, doctors, physical therapists, aides—to the patient's family or guardian. If other people do not know about the bioethical problem, they cannot do anything to help resolve it. In Case Example 7–3, the nurse's aide must tell the doctor that according to his observations, the patient may be able to experience pain. It is essential for the doctor to know this. The doctor may be basing his judgment about the patient on her chart and not on his direct knowledge and examination of her. If the doctor has an office nurse or a medical technician, the aide should talk to them about his concerns as well. If this does not alter the doctor's approach, the aide also needs to communicate his concerns about the patient's potential pain to the patient's mother.

Choose the Appropriate Action

At this point, after the problem is identified, the information gathered, and the communication done, a **choice** needs to be made. Two morals are in conflict. In Case Example 7–3, the moral conflict is between protecting the patient and working with the doctor. Which is more important? On one hand, the aide may be reluctant to anger the physician by insisting that the patient can feel pain, and he may feel that he needs to protect his job by remaining silent. He might reason that by protecting his job, he will be able to do more good in the long run by helping other patients in the future. On the other hand, his patient is in need of protection, and the aide is the one with the knowledge to protect her. In fact, it is the aide's job to protect his patient.

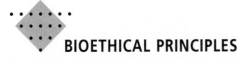

BIOETHICAL PRINCIPLES

To assist medical professionals to make a choice, several moral principles have been identified that are important to health care. All bioethical problems should be evaluated with these principles in mind.

Respect for Autonomy

To be autonomous means to have self-governance or to function independently. "Auto" comes from a Greek word that means "self." Respect for autonomy in bioethical terms means to have respect for the patient to make his own decisions about what is best.

Respect for autonomy is an important principle in bioethics. In the United States there is great respect for individual rights. This respect has been reflected in the law. The law upholds rights of the patient to make decisions about health care. For example, patients are allowed to refuse medical treatment, even if that treatment will save their lives. Patients are not required by law to keep their doctors' appointments and take their medicine, even if that is what the doctors, their families, and their friends think is best for them.

What has been stated in the law is also reflected in current bioethical thought. Under the principle of respect for autonomy, patients should be told the truth, patients should be informed of risks and benefits of treatments, and patients are allowed to refuse treatment.

When analyzing a bioethical problem, consider how the principle of respect for autonomy fits into the puzzle. Is the patient's autonomy

▶ Case Example 7–4

A medical assistant is employed in an oncologist's office. He greets a patient he knows well, a 62-year-old woman with leukemia. Her bloodwork shows that her white blood cell (WBC) count is down. The assistant gives this result to the doctor, who orders an infusion of fresh frozen plasma (FFP). The assistant reminds the doctor that the patient is a Jehovah's Witness, a religious group that refuses all blood products, including FFP, in treatment. The doctor becomes angry. "Just tell her it's medicine that I ordered. Don't tell her it's a blood product. It's not red, so she'll never guess. It's the only thing I have that can help her right now." Should the medical assistant lie to the patient at the request of the doctor? Either he must obey the doctor and lie or refuse to reveal to the patient that the doctor has ordered a blood product for her, or he must disobey the doctor and inform the patient that her treatment is a blood product. His only other option is to leave the office—which will cost him his job and will still not assist the patient. The medical assistant must make a choice.

threatened? Are the options being considered respectful or disrespectful of the patient's autonomy?

For example, in Case Example 7–4, the patient is a Jehovah's Witness. Ignoring her religion shows disrespect for her as an autonomous person who can choose her own religion. Lying shows disrespect because it is assumed that the patient is unable to make decisions about her medical treatment.

Beneficence

Beneficence means doing good or being kind. In bioethical terms, the principle of beneficence means that we as healthcare professionals should always try to help patients and make their situation better. Beneficence is usually the reason many people go into healthcare: they want to help people. It is a strong motivation behind the actions of all healthcare professionals.

When thinking about a bioethical problem, consider whether the actions you are considering will help the patient. For example, in

Case Example 7–1, where the AIDS patient needs extensive dental work, will the dental work help the patient? Yes, it will, because he has an abscessed tooth. Will refusing to do the dental work help the patient? No, because his tooth infection could spread to other parts of his body.

Nonmaleficence

Nonmaleficence means "doing no harm." It is part of a physician's oath to do no harm. In bioethical terms, the principle of nonmaleficence means that healthcare professionals should avoid harming a patient. Nonmaleficence is different but sometimes overlaps with beneficence. **Beneficence means doing good.** In the case of a bioethical dilemma, it is important to make sure that the actions that you are considering do not cause the patient any harm. Nothing you do should ever make the patient worse.

In Case Example 7–3, for instance, where the doctor may do a surgical procedure on a brain-damaged patient without any anesthesia, the principle of nonmaleficence comes into play. Will performing a surgical procedure without anesthesia harm the patient? The answer is it might, if she can feel pain. Of course, the pain may be short term and overall the procedure might help (the principle of beneficence) the patient.

In Case Example 7–2, where the elderly patient asked the aide to lie about how little she had eaten, the principle of nonmaleficence again comes into play. Will lying for the patient harm the patient? Yes, since the patient's lack of nutrition could go unnoticed and result in deterioration, malnutrition, and possibly death.

Integrity of the Health Professional

This principle has to do with the standards of the healthcare profession. What sort of behavior has the profession as a group decided to allow? What behavior is prohibited? All professions have standards, and it is important to know what standards apply to your profession (Case Example 7–5).

This subject brings to mind this question: what actions show respect for human dignity? Lying to a patient or refusing to provide dental care does not respect the dignity of the patient.

▶ Case Example 7–5

A high school student studying in a health professions course at school spends a day following a nurse in her practice in an obstetrics-gynecology clinic. While at the clinic, a classmate patient comes in to be treated and is recognized by the student. The patient is pregnant and is upset and unsure about what to do about her pregnancy. The nurse, with the student watching and listening, spends a lot of time counseling the patient. Later, the health professions student is stopped by a friend in her class. "Hey, I saw you with Didi in the clinic," the friend observes. "What was she in for? Is she pregnant?" Should the health professions student reveal the patient's diagnosis?

Justice

The principle of justice means treating everyone fairly. Distributing health care justly or fairly is a key issue in many ethical debates. Should health care be given to everyone or only those who can pay? Should more health care be given to those who can pay and less to those who cannot? Should large amounts of healthcare money be given to high-tech treatments for dying patients, and should less money be given to preventive care, such as prenatal care and immunizations? Is it fair to charge more for health care for those patients who engage in poor health behaviors such as smoking, eating high-fat foods, and not using their seatbelts?

In this era of high-cost health care, the principle of justice has become an important factor in bioethics. For example, in Case Example 7–1, in which the AIDS patient needs dental care, the principle of justice seems to dictate that the healthcare professional treat him the same as any other patient.

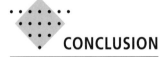

CONCLUSION

Bioethical problems are not easy. Any moral dilemma poses a hard choice between two or more difficult options. At times, the healthcare professional may feel overwhelmed by what may feel like a no-win situation. It is a professional obligation, however, to attempt to determine a solution to the problem to try to serve the patient to the best of the healthcare professional's abilities. Following the steps outlined in this chapter will enable a professional to begin to analyze bioethical problems.

STUDY QUESTIONS

1. What is professional ethics?

2. Define bioethics. Discuss a bioethical dilemma that you have read about or have encountered in practice.

3. Obtain a copy of your code of professional ethics and discuss it with the class.

4. Define and discuss the resolution process for an ethical dilemma.

5. List and define five bioethical principles.

6. Find an ethical case in literature or on the internet and do a case study analysis.

7. Create an ethical dilemma and role play in the class.

REFERENCES

1. Bedell, S. E. (1986). Do not resuscitate orders for critically ill patients in the hospital. *JAMA* 256, 233–237.

2. Lipton, H. L. (1986). DNR decisions in a community hospital. *JAMA,* 256, 1164–1169.

RESOURCES

1. Anronheim, J. C. *Ethics in a Clinical Practice,* 2nd Edition. Gaithersburg: Aspen Publishers, 2000.

2. Beauchamp, T. L. & Childress, J. F. (1994). *Principles of Biomedical Ethics* (4th ed.) New York: Oxford University Press.

3. Beauchamp, T. L. & Walters, L. (1994). *Contemporary issues in bioethics* (4th ed.) Belmont, California: Wadsworth Publishing Co.

4. Cohen C. B. (ed.) (1988). *Casebook on the termination of life-sustaining treatment and the care of dying.* Bloomington, Indiana: Indiana University Press.

5. Crigger, B.-J. (1999). *Cases in Bioethics: Selections from the Hastings Center Report.* (3rd ed.) New York: Bedford Books.

6. The Hastings Center. (1987). *Guidelines on the termination of life-sustaining treatment and the care of the dying.* Briarcliff Manor, New York: The Hastings Center.

7. Howell, J. H., Sale, W. F. & Callahan, D. (Eds.) (2000). *Life choices: A Hastings Center introduction to bioethics. Hastings Center Studies in Ethics* (2nd ed.) Washington, DC: Georgetown University Press.

8. Jonsen, A. R., Veatch, R. M. & Walters, L., (eds.) (2000). *Source book in bioethics: A documentary history.* Washington, DC: Georgetown University Press.

9. Ridley, A. (1998). *Beginning bioethics: A Texas with integrated readings.* New York: Bedford Books.

10. Veatch, R. M. (1999). *The basics of bioethics.* Saddle River, New Jersey: Prentice Hall.

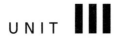

COMMON AREAS
OF LIABILITY
AND LITIGATION

8

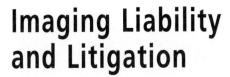

Imaging Liability and Litigation

ARDELE Y. FLOAT, RN, JD

Special Section on Dental Assistant and Hygienist

BRITTA E. LAFONT, RDH, BA, Med and NANCY V. CLINE, RDH, MPH

▶ Key Chapter Concepts

Civil Negligence
Ordinary Negligence
Professional Negligence
Medical Technologist
Ionizing Radiation (X-Rays)
X-Ray Technician
Radiology Technician
Radiology Technologist
Ultrasound Technician
Dental Assistant and Hygienist
Cavitation

▶ Objectives

At the conclusion of this chapter, the reader will have a better understanding of:

1. The liability that arises in allied health professions when using various imaging methods.

2. The common areas of liability for x-ray technicians, radiology technicians and technologists, ultrasound technicians, dental assistants and hygienists, and medical technologists.

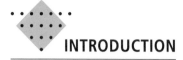

INTRODUCTION

D ental x-rays have become a fairly common and painless experience for most Americans. When your dentist orders x-rays of your teeth, you probably believe there is little risk of injury. Unfortunately, the same technology used to assist diagnosis and treatment can also cause serious injury.

▶ Case Scenario

On March 28, 1985, a female dental patient went to a major medical center dental department for treatment. Twenty x-rays of her mouth were taken using incorrect technique by a student x-ray technician. Immediately following the procedure the patient complained of "burning and itching around her mouth." Her tongue dried up and the skin around her mouth and lips began to blister and peel away [1]. This patient sued the teaching hospital for the negligence of the student x-ray technician during the x-ray procedure. Do you think the x-ray technician's actions were below the standard of care required for members of the profession?

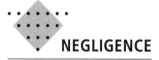

NEGLIGENCE

What does it mean to have a patient name you in a lawsuit for an injury you may have caused while you performed your professional duties? One of the fundamental truths an individual faces when living in an ordered society is responsibility for one's actions. We live under a system of laws that protect the rights of each citizen to seek civil redress in our courts for any injury caused by the negligence of another. The concept of **civil negligence** shares a long history dating back centuries. In our country the law of torts includes an action for **"ordinary negligence"** as well as **"professional negligence."** Ordinary negligence is often defined by the legal scholars as ". . . conduct which involves . . . unreasonable risk of harm . . ." to others [2].

Under the U.S. Constitution, each state is allowed to adopt laws that protect an individual's rights to be free from negligent acts of others. Numerous states have adopted a definition for the professional negligence of persons who have a higher level of education and skill than the ordinary person has. **The essential elements for an action in tort for professional negligence are:**

- **Duty to use due care** [3]
- **Breach of that duty** [4]
- **Detriment to plaintiff** [5]
- **The detriment suffered is an actual (or direct) and legal (or proximate) result of the breach of duty** [6]
- **Damages, the measure of the detriment, is in monetary terms** [7].

Numerous states have adopted a definition for the professional negligence of persons who have a higher level of education and skill than the ordinary person has. For example, in California physicians and other healthcare professionals, under California Civil Code section 1714(a), are subject to medical malpractice actions based on professional negligence standards or due care. "Professional negligence," as defined in the Medical Injury Compensation Reform Act, means a negligent act or omission to act by a healthcare provider in the rendering of professional services, which is the proximate cause of a personal injury or wrongful death, provided that the services are within the scope of services for which the provider is licensed and which are not within any restriction imposed by the licensing agency or licensed hospital [8].

Allied health professions have experienced changes in the legal definition of their level of individual responsibility. In the past, hospitals have borne the burden of defending against the negligence of its employees. Hospital malpractice coverage offered an umbrella of protection for allied health professionals, therefore limiting the individual's exposure to malpractice liability until recently. The professional standard for nurses in malpractice actions has undergone such a change. "As nurses become increasingly visible to the public as interdependent, accountable professionals, the risk of legal responsibility increases." [8a]

The allied health professions that are discussed in this chapter deal with professions using medical technologies as an integral part of their treatment of the patient. We will look at professions that use ionizing radiation (x-ray) to develop images captured on photographic film for purposes of diagnosis and therapy, i.e., radiology technicians and limited licensure technicians [9]. Ultrasound technicians also develop images but use inaudible sound waves in frequency range of approximately 20,000 to 10,000,000,000 cycles/second to outline the shape of various tissues and organs in the body for diagnostic and therapeutic purposes [10]. Dental auxiliaries also work with x-ray medical equipment.

To fully appreciate the type of liability issues that arise with each of the above-named allied health professions, you must look at the history of each profession in terms of state licensure and academic requirements. With an appreciation of the level of required skill, the allied health professional can then evaluate common areas of risk posed to the patient population when negligent care is provided by a subspecialty.

RADIOLOGY TECHNOLOGISTS AND LIMITED LICENSURE TECHNICIANS (X-RAY TECHNICIANS)

Medical technology has become an integral part of the diagnosis and treatment of patients today. Imaging technologies such as x-ray and x-ray computed technology (CAT scan) are relatively new from a historical perspective. CAT scans use x-rays to essentially take computer slices of the body to visualize areas of interest. This technology was first introduced in 1973 and has quickly become an important diagnostic tool.

History of X-Ray Technology

X-ray technology experienced a less dramatic introduction into the hospital setting. **Wilhelm Konrad discovered roentgen rays in 1895** and demonstrated how these roentgen rays could be used to take pictures of internal organs. The technology was initially more of a curiosity than a daily tool for diagnosis until World War I. X-ray technology improved with new x-ray film and portable machines that could treat wounded soldiers on the battlefields. After World War I, x-ray studies emerged as a new specialty in medicine [11].

X-Ray Technicians–Radiology Technicians

Initially, x-ray technology involved just the diagnostic imaging of internal organs, and a new allied health professional called **x-ray technician** was formed to assist physicians. However, as medicine began to treat malignant diseases with small doses of radiation, the duties of the hospital x-ray technician evolved into what is now called the **radiology technician.** An excellent resource that gives a brief history of x-ray technology and the gradual development of radiologic technology from 1944 to the present is the *Health Professions Education Directory* published by the American Medical Association.

The *Health Professions Education Directory* contains information on 47 occupations and their respective accrediting agencies. The directory explains how the profession developed standards of professional practice and selected a national accrediting agency for radiology and radiation therapy educational programs. The national registry, the *American Registry of Radiologic Technologists*, gives examinations for certification [12].

Monitoring of the Professional

Another important function that each state provides to its citizens is the monitoring of healthcare professions to insure quality care. Some states have chosen to closely regulate radiology technicians and limited licensure technicians. Fourteen states do not formally license these professions. For purposes of discussion, California is used as an example of what you may experience if you select to pursue one of these careers.

In California the Department of Health Services, Radiologic Health Branch, began requiring certification for any person administering therapeutic or diagnostic x-rays after July 1, 1971. The state legislature declared that it was in the public's interest to protect its citizens from excessive and improper exposure to ionizing radiation [13]. California established educational standards and developed a state certification procedure that requires applicants to prove completion of specified areas of course study.

Limited Licensure Technologist (X-Ray Technician)

The limited licensure technologist (x-ray technician) has a more limited scope of practice than the radiology technologist does. The x-ray technician only uses ionizing radiation for diagnostic purposes. The x-ray technician has specific training to perform x-rays of the chest, extremities, gastrointestinal (GI), genitourinary (GU), leg-podiatric, skull, or torso-skeletal categories. California licenses x-ray technicians, and the basic program is at least 100 hours of classroom instruction, additional hours in anatomy, physiology, and positioning for taking films of the chest, extremities, GI, GU, leg-podiatric, skull, and torso-skeletal. There are additional clinic hours in each category focusing on quality control consideration issues. These programs are generally 9 months to 1 year, depending upon how many of the subspecialties are completed.

The x-ray technician may just take course work for chest, extremities, and torso-skeletal to enable them to work in offices of orthopedic physicians. Many x-ray technicians are employed in medical offices rather than hospitals. Programs enroll people who have recently graduated from high school; so this is a very attractive career choice for someone interested in entering the job market quickly [14]. Some states also have an approval process for those interested in on-the-job training for x-ray technician [15].

Radiology Technologist

Radiology technologists are usually employed in hospitals and cancer centers to deliver radiation to patients for therapeutic purposes. The training includes the diagnostic use of x-ray as well as the therapeutic application of radiation. California has specific educational requirements that must be satisfied by both the applicant seeking to take the certification examination and the school providing the radiology training [16]. The course of study is at least 455 hours of formal classroom instruction, 15 hours of general radiographic laboratory, 60 hours of physics and radiation protection laboratory, 75 hours of radiotherapy laboratory, and 1,500 hours of supervised clinical education.

Many of these programs are 2-year programs offering an associate of arts degree. There are some 12-month programs offering a certificate, as well as several 4-year programs providing a bachelor of science degree. Information regarding state schools may be found in the *Health Professions Education Directory.*

▶ Case Example 8–1

The American Radiology Technologists (ART), a national organization which gives a certification examination to approved schools, was being offered as sufficient to exempt students from sitting for the state certification examination. In this case the x-ray technicians argued that the state legislature under Health and Safety Code section 25678 (now 107000) allowed for a hearing to determine if ART's education requirements were equivalent to those established by the department. The State Board of Health previously refused to grant recognition to the ART. The x-ray technicians argued that the legislature failed to give adequate standards for the department in reaching its decision to grant reciprocity. The appellate court found that the legislature had provided sufficient guidelines to justify the regulations that required applicants pass the state examination. Therefore, it was a violation of the law for anyone to use diagnostic or therapeutic x-rays on humans in California without passing the state certification examination [17].

States allow out-of-state applicants who have proof of national certification by the American Registry of Radiologic Technologists to sit for the state certification examination. If an applicant is not nationally certified or has lost this certification, the applicant must complete studies in the state to sit for that particular examination. It is important that you determine if there is reciprocity in your state and what is required to practice in the state you have chosen. The issue of reciprocity was litigated by two separate groups of x-ray technicians in California who sought to waive the newly enacted state examination (see Case Example 8–1).

COMMON AREAS OF LIABILITY FOR X-RAY TECHNICIANS OR RADIOLOGY TECHNOLOGISTS

When you consider selecting the profession of x-ray technician or radiology technologist, it is important to understand common areas of liability for these allied health professionals.

Violation of State Statutes

Most of us are too young to remember the use of x-rays in the shoe stores. We now know how harmful excessive exposure to ionizing radiation is to the human cell. This was not as well understood in the 1930s, when it was common practice to fit shoes using x-rays. Some states, such as California, have made it a misdemeanor to use x-rays to help view the bones in the feet for the purpose of fitting shoes [18].

Persons who violate state laws may be subject to both criminal and civil penalties[19]. It is very important for the allied health professional to limit their activities to what is allowed under their certification. Acting beyond the scope of practice can result in being charged with a **misdemeanor and revocation of certification.**

Additionally, states also require additional certification and continuing education for anyone taking mammograms. A certified radiology technologist (CRT) can be found guilty of a **misdemeanor** if working in a mammography clinic without proper certification [20]. You must know what your specific state requires for continued education and additional certifications.

There has been an expansion in the scope of practice of radiology technologists in some parts of the country. Certified radiology technologists are required to follow any new changes in the regulations that affect their profession. For example, trained radiology technologists may start intravenous lines for the sole purpose of administering contrast materials in the upper extremities only [21]. However, CRTs without special training are restricted to only assisting a physician or surgeon in completing an injection to administer contrast materials. The physician must be physically present in the facility and immediately available to respond to any problems that arise. Liability arises if the CRT acts beyond the scope of practice that the law allows.

Prior Criminal Convictions

The states can deny, revoke, or suspend the certification of any person who is found guilty of criminal or unprofessional behavior (e.g., using alcohol or drugs while performing professional duties). The state may also revoke a certification if the person is convicted of a felony or misdemeanor involving moral turpitude that is committed during the performance of radiologic technology duties. This means that, in the interest of public and patient safety, the person may be disciplined if he or she poses a potential threat or harm.

Incompetence or Gross Negligence in Performing Radiologic Technology Functions

State Action Against the CRT

States that regulate radiology technologists may deny an applicant who wishes to sit for the certification exam or suspend or revoke certificates if the radiology technologist's actions fall below the required standard of care of the profession.

Standard of Care

What does it mean to fall below the standard of care? Who decides if someone has endangered a patient? When a state decides to regulate a healthcare profession, the state legislature designates a regulatory body to carry out the specific directions of the legislature. States have different administrative directives, but the general intent is the same—to regulate the allied health professionals who provide radiological services to the public.

The second question is, who decides if a breach of the standard has occurred? The state regulatory body may receive a complaint from an injured patient or a family member. The state may receive a complaint from an employer or fellow employee working with a radiology technologist or x-ray technician. This incident may never result in a formal civil lawsuit being filed for negligence. However, some states revoke a state certificate for incompetence or gross negligence occurring while performing radiologic technology functions [22].

If a formal lawsuit is filed against a certified radiology technologist, the state may decide to investigate the alleged actions of the CRT. This investigation is independent and without regard to the outcome of the civil action. There is a possibility that you may win the civil action for negligence yet still face discipline from the state regulatory body.

CIVIL LITIGATION FOR NEGLIGENCE

On a daily basis, these two professions must provide safe care for all patients receiving treatment. The medical equipment used poses known hazards based upon the fact that radioactive substances cause serious injuries. The following are cases where patients were injured because of the medical equipment.

Radiation Burns

What happens if a patient suffers burns resulting from x-ray treatment? One early case involving the negligence of an x-ray operator conducting a fluoroscopic examination resulted in severe burns to the patient's back. In this case the court reviewed the history of x-rays and determined that an x-ray specialist stood in the same relation to the physician who employed him. This was one of the earliest determinations by a court regarding the standard of care to be applied to x-ray technicians [23].

Seven years later a man sued for injuries that he alleged were due to exposure to excessive radiation. His foot was burned and amputated from 2½ hours of exposure to x-rays. The physician stated it was only a few seconds. Due to the discrepancy, the court left the determination of truthfulness to the jury. In reviewing the evidence, the court found that x-ray burns do occasionally occur in the ordinary course of exposure in spite of the highest diligence and skill to prevent them. Because certain persons are more sensitive than others are and this idiosyncrasy cannot be determined before or during the exposure, the patient assumes the risk [24].

In reviewing the cases, it is apparent that the risk of burns was a real problem in the 1920s. However, 25 years later the same considerations arose in the case of a minor. A 9-year-old boy suffered radiation burns to his heel after receiving x-ray treatments to remove a wart. The court noted that expert testimony revealed that there was no method by which to determine the amount of x-ray a person could take without burning. Again, the expert testimony was that some persons were able to take more x-rays than others, the same way one person may be able to take more sunshine than another without burning [25]. In another case, a patient sued when he suffered severe burns to portions of his head, face, and neck from an x-ray treatment that was given to remove a growth from his ear [26].

Due to the nature of ionizing radiation, the risk of burns has continued to be a problem for patients 100 years after the discovery of Roentgen rays in 1895. Radiation technologists assist physicians in providing radiation cobalt therapy. In one such incident, a hospital and its employee were sued for radiation burns resulting from cobalt therapy under the theory of strict liability. They were found not liable for the professional service rendered [27].

You will remember in the beginning of this chapter that burns were suffered during a dental x-ray procedure and resulted in litigation for negligence[28]. In another case, the court noted that due to the idiosyncrasy of certain persons to x-ray, it would be difficult to know until after the x-ray if they would suffer a burn accident [29].

Falls

X-ray equipment poses a serious risk of harm to the patient if operated in a negligent manner. However, a patient treated in an x-ray department can suffer severe injuries that are unrelated to the medical equipment. In one case, a patient sued for injuries suffered due to falling from a rolling x-ray table. She stated that after the x-ray technician took the ordered x-ray films, she was left unattended on a gurney. She experienced a coughing spasm and fell to the floor [30]. A case with very similar facts 20 years earlier involved a woman left unattended on a gurney while the x-ray technician developed the films. While unattended, she developed a fit of coughing and fell to the floor, suffering spinal injuries [31].

Hospital patients may become faint during an x-ray procedure resulting in liability for those responsible for the patient's safety. In one such case, a patient who had a history of dizzy spells fainted while standing on an x-ray platform and sustained severe injuries. In this case, the radiologist and x-ray technician did not attempt to obtain a clinical history, and the requisition for x-ray had a space for the entry of history but was blank. The court found that both the radiologist and x-ray technician were negligent [32]. Ten years later, a similar case involving an x-ray technician who did not use straps to protect a heavily sedated patient from falling resulted in liability for the hospital. In this case, an expert witness for the injured patient was called to give testimony regarding the training his university provided for the x-ray technician named in the litigation. He stated that if a technologist knew a patient was sedated, then special precautions should be used to prevent injury. He attributed almost 90% of all injuries in the x-ray department to patients falling [33]. Apparently falls continue to be a problem, as shown by the recent case of a patient who fell from an unattended x-ray table [34].

One of the most interesting cases is from California. A radiology technician and numerous physicians and hospital administrators were named in a suit by a family for the death of their mother. The mother fell while being x-rayed, and she was later found to have suffered a life-threatening injury to her cervical spine. The radiology technician explained that while she was positioning the patient to take x-rays of her feet, the woman fell. The mother's sons were both attorneys, and they filed charges against the defendants for breaking their mother's neck, conspiring to conceal the existence of the broken neck, refusing to treat it, intentionally performing useless operations upon their mother to obtain Medicare and MediCal funds, and then attempting to kill their mother to conceal their complicity in causing and concealing the existence of the broken neck [35].

Contrast Materials and Adverse Reactions

Every profession faces the possibility of litigation for mistakes that are the result of careless or improper technique. Patients fall off of x-ray tables, sustain burns or electric shocks from equipment, or even suffer adverse reactions to contrast materials if they are allergic to the dyes used. One case involved the death of a patient receiving an intravenous pyelogram for diagnosing a kidney ailment. An iodine compound called diodrast was used because it is opaque to roentgen rays and can outline the affected parts for diagnostic purposes. Unfortunately, many patients are allergic to the iodine contained in diodrast but that may not be known until a test dose is given. In this case, even though the physician was alerted to symptoms, he chose to treat the initial symptoms and give the remaining lethal dose [36].

As discussed, some states now allow a radiology technologist with additional training to start intravenous lines and to assist the radiologist in giving contrast materials. The hospital does not have to staff a registered nurse in the radiology department; however, it raises potential new areas of liability for the radiology technologist. One such concern was raised in a radiography textbook discussing the changing funding for health care and its impact on the selection of contrast materials. The nonionic agents that were introduced in the 1980s are less likely to stimulate an anaphylactic response such as that which resulted in the death of the mother noted above. These agents are more comfortable for patients but are more expensive. Because of increasing emphasis on hospitals to contain costs, these low-osmolality contrast agents are often only used if the patient has a history of allergy or other physical condition that poses a higher risk. This is unfortunate, because the nonionic agents produce less of the uncomfortable sensation of heat when injected [37].

If any of these accidents do occur, what is the legal standard of negligence for x-ray technicians and radiology technicians? As mentioned earlier, each state defines whether the x-ray technician or radiology technologist's actions are to be held to the standard of ordinary or professional negligence. Often the hospital's level of negligence is being litigated along with whether the employee's actions are covered by the hospital [38] (Case Example 8–2). **Generally, the rule is that the x-ray operator must perform to the same level of skill as others with similar training and work experience in similar localities [39].** However, some courts have applied a higher standard of care required of physicians and surgeons to the nonphysician x-ray

---

▶ Case Example 8–2

At approximately 3:30 a.m. on August 2, 1993, a 75-year-old patient tumbled coming from her bathroom and fell, striking her head. She was unable to get up and lay on the floor until approximately 8:00 a.m., when a home health aide came to her home for her daily visit. Emergency medical services arrived and transported the patient to the hospital. After treatment in the emergency room, she was admitted as a patient. Two of the patient's friends went to the hospital. She was taken for skull x-rays. When she returned, the x-ray technologist said that there had been "a little accident." He stated, "the x-ray plate fell on her head." He showed where it had fallen on the patient's head. One of the friends pushed back the patient's hair and saw a blue mark on the left side of her forehead. The patient told her friend that the technicians were "cutting up" when the x-ray cartridge slipped and fell on her head. The patient's internist said that he received a "panic call" from a nurse who found a large acute subdural hematoma. Surgery was performed to evacuate the hematoma. The patient died on August 16, 1993. Her sons brought a wrongful death suit against the hospital. A jury found for the plaintiffs. The hospital appealed.

operator because of the high degree of skill and care in the use of x-rays [40]. (To protect your license and avoid litigation, you should follow the national standards of care for your specialty and profession.)

Unknown Future Injury

The history of the use of x-ray therapy has numerous cases where the new technology caused unanticipated injury. Fluoroscope operators exhibited increased rates of lethal skin carcinomas. There was an increased rate of radiation-induced leukemia with radiologists and their assistants. Pregnant mothers receiving pelvic radiotherapy gave birth to infants with severe mental retardation. Newborns given radiation therapy to shrink the thymus gland as preventative therapy to prevent sudden infant death syndrome (SIDS) later developed thyroid cancer. Treatments for unwanted hair were initially success-ful, but radiation dermatitis and skin cancers appeared later. Studies have also shown a link with lung cancer for men given radiotherapy for ankylosing spondylitis [41].

We now understand the risk to the developing fetus of genetic damage from radiation. There is concern for potential genetic dam-age to the ovum or sperm before conception resulting in injury to the fetus. A recent study of women who were exposed as children to ionizing radiation from diagnostic radiography showed an associa-tion with low birthweight in their offspring [42]. In hindsight, it is now clear that the risks of radiation were not fully appreciated in the early years of radiation therapy. With the increased applications for ionizing radiation in the future there may well be yet unidentified risks resulting in litigation.

ULTRASOUND TECHNICIANS

Hospitals and clinics throughout the country utilize sonography (ultrasound) to visualize internal organs with sound waves. At this time, no state has regulated the use of ultrasound on the public because sonography does not use ionizing radiation. This means that no state agency is responsible for overseeing this profession. At this point, the profession regulates itself and has set up educational requirements and professional standards and guidelines. Educational programs that meet the standards are recommended for accreditation to the Commission on Accreditation of Allied Health Education Programs by the Joint Review Committee on Accreditation of Allied Health Education Programs by the Joint Review Committee on Education in Diagnostic Medical Sonography. Programs can be 1 to 4 years depending on the degree of specialty. The American Registry of Diagnostic Medical Sonographers (ARDMS) offers to this allied health specialty three credentials and serves as both a certifying body as well as a disciplinary board [43].

The three credentials provided by ARDMS are registered diagnostic cardiac sonographer (RDCS), registered diagnostic medical sonographer (RDMS), and registered vascular technologist (RVT). Hospitals and clinics that provide this service are responsible for selecting adequately trained sonographers. One way that the profession is passively regulated is through financial reimbursements. The Health Care Financing Administration (HCFA) has recommended that all state Medicare carriers require the sonographers to be credentialed in vascular technology as either a registered vascular technologist or a registered cardiovascular technologist [44].

POTENTIAL AREAS OF LIABILITY FOR ULTRASOUND TECHNICIANS

Violation of State Statutes

We know that no state has chosen to regulate this practice. Therefore, any disciplinary action will be provided by an employer, an ARDMS certifying body, or civil litigation.

Prior Criminal Convictions

Some states can revoke the certification of the x-ray technician or radiology technologist for criminal acts that were committed while performing professional duties. The national registry, ARDMS, has an even broader disciplinary policy. The certificate holder may lose certification not only for crimes which occurred while providing medical services, but also if it is deemed to be directly related to public health [45].

Incompetence or Gross Negligence in Performing Radiologic Technology Functions

ARDMS can impose sanctions. Because there is no state regulation of this profession, ARDMS has become the agency that receives complaints about any possible violation of ARDMS standards by its certified members [46].

CIVIL AND CRIMINAL LITIGATION

During the first 100 years of using ionizing radiation, we learned that there are many unknown risks that will only be appreciated with time. Based upon this knowledge, an international group was formed in Vienna, Austria, in June 1969 to look at the application of ultrasound techniques in biological and medical research and to promote cooperation. **The World Federation for Ultrasound in Medicine and Biology (WFUMB) was formed as a nonprofit scientific organization, and one of its goals is to encourage research in the field and share the knowledge within the international medical community.** Practice groups were formed to deal with areas of concern such as thermal bioeffects and cavitation to attempt to reach a policy statement for approved safety parameters.

In 1991, the WFUMB met in Hornbaek, Denmark, to evaluate the research on the biological effects on tissues from the heat generated during ultrasound. In the following year, the WFUMB published its recommendations regarding thermal effects and safety guidelines. In 1992, the focus of the symposium was on the nonthermal effects such as cavitation and acoustic radiation and fluid streaming, as well as the nonthermal threshold [47].

Burns

The WFUMB identified the risk of burning soft tissue/bone interfaces with some Doppler diagnostic equipment. A few of the recommendations are to limit the time for each beam pass and keep the output power as low as possible. Because of the concern for fetal injury with obstetric ultrasound, the recommendation is to limit the duration of exposure and avoid any unnecessary examinations if the mother has a fever because the risk to the fetus is increased [48].

Nonthermal Effects

Numerous animal studies have demonstrated the risk of **cavitation, which is the formation of air bubbles in a fluid medium**. One recent study looked at the destructive effect of inertial cavitation on human platelets when contrast agents were used to enhance the ultrasound imaging. Obviously, these studies were not conducted on human subjects, but the WFUMB has issued current safety guidelines covering the use of contrast agents and power output range [49].

Actions Outside the Scope of Practice

Because this is a relatively new profession, there is little relevant case law involving negligence of ultrasound technicians. However, one case in California raises some interesting public policy concerns regarding the conduct of an ultrasound technician. In this case, a pregnant woman was seen in an emergency room for injuries suffered from a fall at a movie theater. The emergency room physician ordered an obstetrical and upper-right-quadrant ultrasonic imaging examination. The ultrasound technician would not allow the patient to have her mother or boyfriend present in the examination room. The door to the examination room was closed. Following completion of the examination, the ultrasound technician offered to discover the sex of the baby for the young mother. She consented to the examination, but later that day she realized that his actions were improper. He used the ultrasound equipment to molest her. She sued the hospital and the ultrasound technician for professional negligence, battery, and intentional and negligent infliction of emotional harm. **The ultrasound technician plead no contest to a felony charge of sexual molestation.**

The California Supreme Court ultimately heard this case. A majority of the court decided to relieve the hospital of liability for the inappropriate actions of its employee. The majority reasoned that the technicians' conduct was beyond the scope of his employment as a matter of law, that the sexual conduct and emotions were not work related, and that the hospital could not reasonably foresee that this conduct would result from his work duties or the nature of his employment. The court reasoned that the technician "simply took advantage of solitude with a naive patient to commit an assault for reasons unrelated to his work." Based upon procedural grounds, two dissenting opinions were written which is an example of how our court system presents differing views [50].

Another noncriminal penalty that could be faced by the offender in this type of situation is from the WFUMB. The conduct could be found to be detrimental to the honor or interests of the federation, resulting in the technician's being expelled [51].

The ultrasound profession is still new, and ultrasound imaging is becoming an increasingly valuable diagnostic tool in medicine. One new sonographic technique is called **interventional ultrasound, which uses ultrasound to guide a needle for diagnostic and therapeutic purposes.** One application is in obtaining tissue biopsies of the breast or prostate to diagnose cancer. Another technique is to use an ultrasound-guided needle to deliver x-ray contrast agents to a specific hollow organ or tubular structure for diagnostic purposes. The possibilities of an exciting professional career may definitely be found in ultrasound imaging. The accompanying liability will undoubtedly surface with the advent of expanded applications, which will require diligence on the part of the ultrasound technician to keep abreast of the research [52].

DENTAL AUXILIARIES

Another professional who takes x-rays of patients is the dental-related professional. The dental assistant and dental hygienist are two professionals who are now routinely found in a dental office. The **dental assistant,** who receives 2 years of on-the-job training or attends a 9-month course, may sit for national certification. The **dental hygienist** educational programs are generally a 2-year associate's degree or a 4-year bachelor's degree.

LEGAL AND ETHICAL ISSUES IN DENTAL HYGIENE

The profession of dental hygiene is in a state of constant evolution. Change is driven by factors such as the results of research and scientific discovery, advances in technology, developments in the managed care industry, and the revision of laws governing the practice of dental hygiene and dentistry. Additionally, the actual practice of dental hygiene can vary a great deal from one state to another in terms of duties, supervision, and regulation. However, dental hygienists across the United States and around the world share a common bond. By definition, "the dental hygienist is a licensed primary healthcare professional, oral health educator, and clinician who, as a co-therapist, provides preventive, educational, and therapeutic services supporting total health for the control of oral diseases and the promotion of oral health" [53].

Education and Continuing Education

Dental hygienists are educated in a variety of settings, including community colleges, 4-year colleges, and dental schools. The minimum length of a dental hygiene program is 2 academic years following high school graduation.

Practice Settings

The vast majority of dental hygienists with associate's degrees and baccalaureate degrees work in private solo or group dental practices under the supervision of a dentist. Only in Colorado is it legal for a hygienist to treat patients as an independent practitioner in a separate facility.

In addition to private practice, there are other settings in which dental hygienists find employment. Dental hygienists with associate's degrees generally work in private practice. In many cases, alternative work settings may be open only to those who hold a baccalaureate degree.

Professional Associations

The American Dental Hygienists Association (ADHA) was founded in 1923 and has approximately 35,000 members. ADHA publishes the *Journal of Dental Hygiene, Access and Education Update.* The association is a source of information on state practice acts, expanded dental hygiene functions, educational programs, and legislative issues. It is the voice of organized dental hygiene in areas of health policy and maintains a presence in Washington, D.C. ADHA through its Institute for Oral Health provides scholarships to dental hygiene students throughout the country.

The National Dental Hygienists Association (NDHA) was founded in 1932 to address the special problems and needs of the minority dental hygienist. In addition to promoting the art and science of dental hygiene, the NDHA has as its goals expanding continuing education and employment opportunities and facilitating student recruitment and scholarship. The NDHA offers scholarships to deserving minority students each year.

Other Legal Issues

Liability insurance protects personal and professional assets in the event of professional liability in a malpractice lawsuit. Traditionally, dental hygienists have not been the target of dental malpractice lawsuits. However, if the hygienist is sued for malpractice, the dentist's liability insurance may not cover him or her.

Standard of care is a measure of the care that a reasonable and sensible person would use in the same situation. Legally, members of the profession determine this (see Case Examples 8–3 through 8–5). The actual care that is given to a patient will depend upon the type of procedure being performed. As previously mentioned, the duties of the dental hygienist may vary a great deal from state to state, as will

---

▶ Case Example 8–3

Infection Control Procedures: You are working as a hygienist in a very successful general dentistry practice. The full-time employees all receive a very generous bonus if monthly goals are met. Everyone is extremely cost-conscious because when supply costs are controlled, it is easier to meet the monthly goal. You are all for controlling costs, but you realize that disposable items like suction tips, prophy angles, and air/water syringe tips are being re-used on patients. You are told, "Relax, we put them in cold sterilization overnight. We can't just throw them away; they are perfectly good. Why should we waste money?" Everyone agrees with this statement except you. You know that your state's dental practice act specifically mentions this issue and prohibits the re-use of single-use supplies. What should you do?

▶ Case Example 8–4

Failure to Refer Patients to a Specialist: You have been with the same office for the last 7 years. You work in a practice owned by a father and son team of dentists. You really enjoy the work and the pay is great. Both of your bosses are easygoing and the patients just love them! Both dentists, who have often complimented your work, respect you. You do a lot of the root planing of patients in your office as an initial therapy. Then you usually send them to a periodontist if the pockets persist. Lately, both dentists have been reluctant to refer patients to the periodontist. Four months ago they attended a seminar on maintaining periodontal patients in a general dentistry practice. Now they want to keep the patients in the office and have you treat the patient with more root planing, irrigation, and other local chemotherapeutics. You are uncomfortable with this new role because you feel that many of the patients have problems beyond what you are able to manage. Both dentists tell you that it will just take a little time to get used to it and they know you will do a great job. What should you do?

the procedures being performed by dental hygienists. The list below will serve to illustrate the standard of care as applied to a particular procedure.

The typical dental hygiene procedure is referred to as a recall appointment, a maintenance appointment, a prophylaxis, or a "proxy." In general, the following tasks should be accompanied at each prophylaxis appointment:

- Complete or update the medical history with the patient
- Take and record the blood pressure of the patient
- Take and develop any necessary radiographs
- Perform an assessment of the head and neck, including the oral cavity
- Perform an examination of the periodontal issues (to include a recording of clinical attachment levels at least once per year or more often if major changes have occurred)

▶ Case Example 8–5

Nondiagnosis of dental disease: You have just started work at a new office. The previous hygienist, Sally, was with the practice for 18 years and everyone misses her. The patients are all disappointed to see that she is gone. The dentist is always saying that you will be fine if you just do things the way she did them. However, as you see more of the patients, you realize that Sally was not recording clinical attachment levels on each patient. In many charts, you do not even find evidence of yearly probing depths. As you begin to perform examinations and record clinical attachment levels on all patients, you encounter resistance from both the patients and the dentist. They do not understand why it takes you longer than the 30 minutes it used to take Sally. Worse than that, you are disturbed by your findings. The overwhelming majority of patients are exhibiting signs of significant periodontal involvement. When you discuss this with the patients, some do not believe you and say, "If I have so many problems, then why didn't Sally tell me. She was my hygienist for many years. She knew my mouth better than you do." The dentist grumbles that what you are doing is going to scare all of the patients away. Other patients become angry at you and at Sally: "What do you mean I have gum disease? I have never missed an appointment to get my teeth cleaned! Are you saying the other girl wasn't doing her job? Why didn't the dentist catch it? Who is going to pay for all this treatment you say that I need?" How can you answer these questions without making the situation worse? Should you keep your mouth shut?

- Perform an examination of the teeth to identify areas in need of additional dental care
- Evaluate oral hygiene and give oral hygiene instructions
- Remove the supragingival and subgingival deposits
- Polish the teeth as indicated
- Give a professional fluoride treatment, if indicated

- Document all findings, procedures performed, and any patient concerns.

Most of the areas of litigation with this profession deal with acting outside of the legal scope of practice, such as the dental assistant performing duties to be performed by a dental hygienist. The dental assistant and dental hygienist may operate dental radiographic equipment if they have passed the state examination.

All the risks posed by the use of x-rays discussed earlier apply to dental x-rays. Consider the case scenario describing the dental patient who suffered severe burns to the mouth and tongue due to incorrect technique. Based upon your own experience and the knowledge you now have of the known risks, do you think the technician's actions posed an unreasonable risk of harm to this patient?

CONCLUSION

The professions that deal with medical imaging are relatively new in the medical field, and many of the risks are still not fully appreciated. The largest number of litigated cases arise out of the field of radiography, which is understandably due to the very nature of the Roentgen rays discovered 100 years ago. Medical practitioners have some appreciation of the dangers from radiation, but ultrasound therapy is still in a research stage, evaluating what the degree of biological hazards may exist from ultrasound imaging. Certainly, the future will prove quite exciting for anyone considering these allied health professions.

PERTINENT POINTS

1. CAT scans use x-rays to essentially take computer slices of the body to visualize areas of interest and was first introduced in 1973.
2. William Konrad discovered roentgen rays in 1895 and demonstrated how these roentgen rays could be used to take pictures of internal organs.
3. The *Health Professions Education Directory* contains information on 47 occupations and their respective accrediting agencies.

4. The x-ray technician uses ionizing radiation for diagnostic purposes.
5. Radiology technologists are usually employed in hospitals and cancer centers to deliver radiation to patients for therapeutic purposes.
6. Common areas of liability for x-ray technicians and radiology technologists include the following:
   a. Violation of state statutes
   b. Prior criminal convictions
   c. Incompetence or gross negligence
   d. Radiation burns
   e. Falls
   f. Contrast materials adverse reactions.
7. Sonography (ultrasound) is used to visualize internal organs with sound waves.
8. Common areas of malpractice litigation regarding dental hygienists include the following:
   a. Failure to treat problems related to temporomandibular joint syndrome
   b. Failure to diagnose, refer, or treat periodontal condition
   c. Failure to obtain informed consent
   d. Failure to identify and protect a person with a medically compromising condition, such as a heart murmur
   e. Failure to maintain infection control
   f. Failure to maintain proper documentation
   g. Incorrect history taking.

STUDY QUESTIONS

1. What is ordinary negligence?

2. When were roentgen rays discovered and by whom? What were the rays used for in medicine?

3. What is the scope of practice for the x-ray technician?

4. What are four common areas of liability for x-ray technicians and radiology technologists?

5. What is the role of the ultrasound technician?

6. What are the potential areas of liability for the ultrasound technician?

7. What is the role of the dental assistant and dental hygienist?

8. What are the potential "danger zones" of liability for the dental assistant and dental hygienist?

REFERENCES

1. Sosunova v. Regents of the University of California, 11 Cal.Rptr.2d 130,8 Cal.App.4th 1166 (1992).
2. Prosser, W. L., & X. Keton (1984). *On the law of torts: Negligence: Standard of conduct* (5th ed.) (section 31, p. 169). St. Paul: West Publishing Co.
3. California Civil Code sections 1714(a), 3333.
4. California Civil Code sections 3333.
5. California Civil Code sections 3281, 21822, 3333.
6. California Civil Code section 3333.
7. California Civil Code section 3281, 3333.
8. Medical Injury Compensation Reform Act, California Civil Code section 1714 Cal. (Stats. 1975, 2d Ex Sess, chs. 12).
8a. Kjervik, D. K. (Ed.) (1998). Editorial. *Journal of Nursing Law, 5,* 5.
9. *Taber's cyclopedic medical dictionary* (13th ed., 1973) (pp. 1–6). Philadelphia: WB Saunders.
10. *Taber's cyclopedic medical dictionary* (13th ed., 1973) (p. U-3). Philadelphia: WB Saunders.
11. Howell, J. D. (1991). Diagnostic technologies: X-rays, electrocardiograms and CAT scans. *Southern California Law Review 1991, 65,* 529, 533, 536.
12. Donini-Lenhoff, F. (Ed.) (1998). Radiology technology. *Health professions education directory 1998-1999* (26th ed.) (pp. 270–277). Chicago: American Medical Association.
13. California Health and Safety Code section 11484.
14. Title 17 of the California Code of Regulations, subchapter 4.5 Radiologic Technology, section 30424.
15. California Health and Safety Code section 30428.
16. California Health and Safety Code sections 30420–30427.
17. Antoine v. Department of Public Health, 33 Cal.App.3d 215, 108 Cal.Rptr. 689 (1973).
18. California Health and Safety Code section 10699.
19. California Health and Safety Code section 107075.
20. California Health and Safety Code section 106965.
21. California Health and Safety Code section 106985.
22. California Health and Safety Code section 107070(b).
23. Runyan v. Goodrum, 228 S.W. 397, 147 Ark. 481, 13 A.L.R. 1403 (1921).
24. Ballance v. Dunnington, 241 Mich. 383, 217 N.W. 329 (1928).
25. Nance v. Hitch, 238 N.C. 1, 76 S.E.2d 461 (1953).
26. Emrie v. Tice, 174 Kan. 739, 258 P.2d 332 (1953).
27. Nevauex v. Park Place Hospital, Inc., 656 S.W.2d 923 (1993).
28. Sosunova v. Regents of the University of California, 11 Cal.Rptr.2d 130, 8 Cal.App.4th 1166 (1992).

29. Stemons v. Turner, 274 Pa. 228, 117 A. 822, 26 A.L.R. 727 (1922).
30. Garnet v. Central Valley General Hospital, 50 Cal.App.4th 797, 57 Cal.Rptr.2d 894 (1996).
31. Gopaul v. Herrick Memorial Hospital, 38 Cal.App.3d 1002, 113 Cal.Rptr. 811 (1974).
32. Favalora v. Aetna Casualty and Surety Co., 144 So.2d 544 (La.App. 1962).
33. Albritton v. Bossier City Hospital Commission, 271 So.2d 353 (1972).
34. Bellamy v. Central Valley General Hospital, 50 Cal.App.4th 797, 57 Cal.Rptr.2d 894 (1996).
35. Mann v. Cradcchiolo, 38 Cal.3d 18, 694 P.2d 1134, 210 Cal.Rptr. 762 (1985).
36. Synder v. Pontaleo, 143 Conn. 290, 122 A.2d 21 (1956).
37. Ehrlich, R. A., McCloskey, E. D., & Daly, J. A. (1999). Contrast media and special imaging techniques. In J. Rowland (Ed.), *Patient care in radiography* (5th ed.) (pp. 268–269). Location: Mosby.
38. Bellamy v. Central Valley General Hospital, 50 Cal.App.4th 797, 57 Cal.Rptr.2d 894(1996); Gopaul v. Herrick Memorial Hospital, 38 Cal.App.3d 1002, 113 Cal. Rptr. 811; Flowers v. Torrance Memorial Hospital, 8 Cal.4th 992, 884 P.2d 142, 35 Cal.Rptr.2d 685.
39. Ballance v. Dunnington, 241 Mich. 383, 217 N.W. 329(1928); Nance v. Hitch, 238 N.C. 1, 76 S.E.2d 461.
40. Runyan v. Goodrum, 147 Ark. 481, 228 S.W. 397(1921); Holt v. Ten Broeck, 134 Minn. 458, 159 N.W. 1073.
41. Miller, R.W. (1995). Delayed effects of external radiation exposure: A brief history. *Radiation Research, 144*(2), 160–165.
42. Goldberg, M. S., Mayo, N. E., Levy, A. R., et al. (1998). Adverse reproductive outcomes among women exposed to low levels of ionizing radiation from diagnostic radiography for adolescent idiopathic scoliosis. *Epidemiology, 3,* 271–278.
43. Commission on Accreation of Allied Health Education Programs: Standards and Guidelines for Diagnostic Medical Sonographer. Essentials/Standards initially adopted in 1979; revised 1987, 1996; Overview of the ARDMS home page Web cite Overview of the ARDMS www.ardms.org/overview.htm.
44. ARDMS: Medicare, Vascular Reimbursement and You, Health Care Financing Administration policy directive. ARDMS generated information sheet 1998.
45. ARDMS: Standing Policy and Procedures. June 28, 1997. ARDMS 2.6.4.1.5.
46. ARDMS: Standing Policy and Procedures. June 28, 1997. ARDMS 2.6.6.
47. World Federation for Ultrasound in Medicine and Biology (1998). Constitution preamble. *Ultrasound in Medicine and Biology, 24*(7), 931–944.
48. WFUMB 1996 Kloster-Banz Symposium (1998). WFUMB symposium on safety of ultrasound in medicine recommendations on the safe use of ultrasound. *Ultrasound in Medicine and Biology, 24*(supplement), xv–xvi.
49. WFUMB 1996 Kloster-Banz Symposium (1998). WFUMB symposium on safety of ultrasound in medicine recommendations on the safe use of ultrasound. *Ultrasound in Medicine and Biology, 24*(supplement), xv–xvi.
50. Lisa M. v. Henry Mayo Newhall Memorial Hospital, 12 Cal.4th 291, 907 P.2d 358, 48 Cal.Rptr.2d 510 (1995).
51. World Federation for Ultrasound in Medicine and Biology; Preface and Constitution (1998). *Ultrasound in Medicine and Biology, 933 24*(7), 931–944.
52. Holm, H. H. (1998). Interventional ultrasound in Europe. *Ultrasound in Medicine and Biology, 24*(6), 779–791.
53. Donini-Lenhoff, F. (Ed.) (1998). Dental-related occupations. *Health professions education directory 1998-1999* (26th ed.) (pp. 89–119). Chicago: American Medical Association.

9

Administrative and Medical Record Liability and Litigation

KATHLEEN M. GIALANELLA, RN, JD

▶ **Objectives**

At the conclusion of the chapter, the reader should have a better understanding of:

1. The importance of protecting a patient's right to privacy.

2. The "need to know" rule.

3. The difference between invasion of privacy and breach of confidentiality.

4. The types of discrimination that can result from the inappropriate release of patient information.

5. Four types of patient information that require heightened protection.

6. Computer safety measures that can be taken to protect patient information.

7. The circumstances that force a facility to refuse to respond to a subpoena duces tecum.

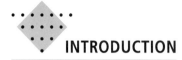

INTRODUCTION

There are many potential ethical dilemmas and legal pitfalls faced by individuals who, because of the nature of their jobs, have access to and/or are responsible for maintaining patient healthcare records. Whether you are a health information technologist or administrator, a medical assistant, a medical custodian, or a medical record transcriptionist, you have access to and control of sensitive patient information. It does not matter what type of healthcare facility employs you. If such information is inappropriately accessed or released, there may be legal ramifications.

▶ Case Scenario

Ester Leaven is a health information administrator at North Island Medical Center. David Farmer, the hospital's vice president of human resources, approaches her. Mr. Farmer requests that Ms. Levin provide him with a printout of certain healthcare records pertaining to Dr. Robert Lewis. Dr. Lewis is employed as a surgical resident at the medical center and was recently hospitalized there. Rumor has it that Dr. Lewis is homosexual and may have tested positive for human immunodeficiency virus (HIV) while hospitalized.

Ms. Levin knows from her training in health information management that information about patients who are HIV positive or diagnosed with acquired immunodeficiency syndrome (AIDS) must be carefully protected. Ms. Levin does not think it appropriate to provide the requested information to Mr. Farmer. Although Mr. Farmer is responsible for hospital personnel, he has never before personally requested hospital records from the patient records department. Ms. Levin asks Mr. Farmer if he has a signed consent form from Dr. Lewis. Mr. Farmer states he does not need one as he is the director of human resources and Dr. Lewis is an employee. Ms. Levin is afraid that if she refuses to provide the requested information she could be disciplined or even lose her job. What should she do?

Failure to adhere to the principles discussed below can lead to legal liability for both the individual who inadvertently or deliberately accesses or releases confidential patient information and the health-care facility for which the responsible individual works.

HEALTHCARE RECORD LIABILITY

Why should you be so concerned about maintaining the confidentiality of a patient record? Our legal system provides each individual with the right of privacy that includes a patient's right to expect that the healthcare record will remain confidential. This right is derived from common law and constitutional law. There are reported legal decisions that uphold a patient's right of privacy, as well as federal and state statutes and regulations that protect this right. For example, hospital regulations in New Jersey require such acute care facilities to have "a medical records department with the primary responsibility of maintaining medical records for all inpatients treated at the hospital" [1].

Protections such as these are necessary to insure a patient's right of privacy and prevent emotional distress from the humiliation and embarrassment of an unauthorized disclosure. Such protections also are necessary because, at times, an individual's health history leads to discrimination on the job, in school, or when applying for certain types of insurance, primarily health and life insurance.

RIGHT OF PRIVACY AND CONSENT

The right of privacy, however, is not absolute. One obvious exception to a facility's policy of nondisclosure is a patient's **consent** to the release of healthcare information. Such consent may be given for a variety of reasons. A patient may wish to provide another healthcare provider or facility with healthcare history in order to receive appropriate treatment. In addition, a patient usually is required to consent to the release of records to the health insurance carrier or managed care company in order to obtain healthcare benefits. Often, healthcare providers are required to disclose certain patient information to governmental authorities. For example, state departments of health require that certain communicable diseases, such as tuberculosis, be promptly reported to the appropriate authorities. In various states the information submitted must contain identifying information for the person diagnosed unless the patient is tested in one of a limited number of testing sites within the state that offer state-mandated anonymous testing.

Under these types of circumstances, a state's interest in protecting the health, safety, and welfare of the public from the threat of communicable diseases outweighs the individual patient's right of privacy. Patient information that is necessary to provide appropriate patient care can be shared between and among treating healthcare providers within the same facility, but such information must not go beyond those who have a **need to know.** For example, a treating physician may order a dietary consultation for his diabetic patient who is about to be discharged from the hospital. The nutritionist is permitted access to the patient record in order to obtain certain information and make an entry regarding the consultation but is not permitted access to a record pertaining to a prior hospitalization of the same patient for a mental illness. Patient records also can be subpoenaed under certain circumstances. If the subpoena is valid, the patient's records must be released.

VIOLATIONS OF PATIENT'S RIGHT OF PRIVACY

If an exception for disclosure does not exist and a patient's record is inappropriately released or accessed, that patient's right to privacy is violated. Claims against healthcare workers for **negligence** and/or **quasi-intentional torts** can follow (Box 9–1). **Invasion of privacy** and **breach of confidentiality** are the most common quasi-intentional torts alleged in lawsuits dealing with the inappropriate disclosure of patient information. "Quasi" means "resembling". This type of tort is based on speech. [Defamation in the form of libel or slander is also a

---

BOX 9–1 • QUASI-INTENTIONAL TORTS

- Invasion of privacy
- Breach of confidentiality

quasi-intentional tort.] [2]. **Invasion of privacy** occurs when someone who has no right to access a patient's healthcare record does so anyway, thereby intruding upon the private concerns of the patient. **Breach of confidentiality** occurs when someone who has legitimate access to health information about a patient shares it with others who have no reason to know. For example, in *Pierce v. Caday* [3], a patient sued her healthcare provider for failure to protect her confidential information from disclosure. The healthcare provider's employees had access to the information and discussed it with others. Although the patient's lawsuit was unsuccessful, it demonstrates that such litigation occurs and affects employees of healthcare providers such as health information management administrators and technicians, medical assistants, medical transcriptionists, and medical secretaries.

Other examples of the legal theories used in liability cases for improper disclosure of patient records are set forth in *Estate of Behringer v. Princeton Medical Center* [4] and *Fairfax Hospital v. Curtis* [5]. In the *Behringer* case, Dr. Behringer, a physician with surgical privileges at Princeton Medical Center and who was also a patient, sued for damages resulting from the medical center and its employees breach of the duty to protect the confidentiality of his diagnosis. In June 1987, Dr. Behringer became ill and was admitted to the medical center for treatment. Part of Dr. Behringer's medical work-up included a bronchoscopy and a blood test for HIV. He tested positive for HIV and the bronchoscopy confirmed the presence of pneumocystis carinii pneumonia (PCP), a common condition found in AIDS patients. These two findings led to a diagnosis of AIDS. The treating physician advised Dr. Behringer of the diagnosis. Thereafter, Dr. Behringer was discharged from the hospital to be treated at home. He was concerned that his diagnosis would become general knowledge—a concern that was not unfounded.

Once home, Dr. Behringer received numerous phone calls from physicians at the medical center. The physicians were not his treating physicians and had no reason to know his diagnosis, although it was clear that they did. Approximately one month after his hospitalization, Dr. Behringer returned to his medical practice, but it was evident that many of his patients had become aware of his diagnosis and his practice began to deteriorate. He lost patients and employees, and his surgical privileges at the hospital were canceled when the chief of nursing told the president of the medical center about Dr. Behringer's diagnosis. Although Dr. Behringer wished to continue performing surgery, he was not allowed to do so. He managed to continue an office practice until his death approximately 2 years later.

Prior to his death, he filed a lawsuit against the medical center and some of its employees. The lawsuit alleged, among other things, that the defendants breached their duty to maintain the confidentiality of Dr. Behringer's diagnosis. The court agreed. Although the court recognized the **need to know exception** to the general rule of confidentiality of patient information, it was clear that the boundaries of the exception had been violated as a result of several factors. The hospital's laboratory had failed to take adequate steps to maintain the confidentiality of the diagnostic test results. In addition, the hospital was negligent as the custodian of patient charts. It failed to take certain steps to limit access and maintain the confidentiality of the records. Although the medical center instructed its employees that medical records were confidential, it was not enough. The medical center knew that most of its staff could access any patient chart with or without authorization. The court found this unacceptable.

In *Fairfax Hospital v. Curtis,* a patient sued a hospital and two of its employees for compensatory and punitive damages. Ms. Curtis claimed her confidential medical records were improperly released to third parties without her consent. The trial court awarded her $100,000.00, and the defendants appealed. The Supreme Court of Virginia upheld the award.

The facts of the case are as follows: Ms. Curtis was a patient at Fairfax Hospital where she received prenatal care and eventually gave birth to a child. During her treatment, she provided certain information about herself to the healthcare providers. The court did not specify the nature of the medical information Mr. Curtis provided (apparently to protect Ms. Curtis from further disclosure of confidential information), but it stated "the medical records contained very personal information about plaintiff's medical history before and after her pregnancy" (*Fairfax Hospital v. Curtis* at 644). After the birth, the child suffered cardiopulmonary arrest and died. Ms. Curtis, as the representative of the child's estate, filed a malpractice claim against the hospital. After receiving notice of the claim, the hospital released a copy of Ms. Curtis' medical records to the attorney it had retained to defend the claim. That attorney, in turn, released the records to a defendant nurse in the malpractice case.

The defendants argued that Ms. Curtis' medical records were properly disclosed because they were at issue in the malpractice case. The court disagreed because at the time Ms. Curtis' records were released by the hospital, it was the deceased child's medical condition that was at issue, not the mother's medical condition. The court determined that releasing such information without the patient's consent is a **tort.**

"[A] healthcare provider owes a duty of reasonable care to the patient. Included within that duty is the healthcare provider's obligation to preserve the confidentiality of information about the patient, which was communicated to the healthcare provider during the course of treatment. Indeed, confidentiality is an integral aspect of the relationship between a healthcare provider and a patient and, often, to give the healthcare provider the necessary information to provide proper treatment, the patient must reveal the most intimate aspects of his or her life to the healthcare provider during the course of treatment."

Fairfax Hospital v. Curtis at 644

Patients have a right to assume that if they share information with their healthcare provider, it remains confidential and is only shared for the purposes of assuring appropriate treatment and proper recordation.

Healthcare facilities are required to implement meaningful **restrictions on access to patient records.** It is not enough to merely instruct all employees about the confidentiality of patient information. Healthcare facilities must actively limit or prevent access in keeping with the need to know rule. Failure to act accordingly can result in serious harm to the patient, as it did in Dr. Behringer's case. Also, those with access to patient charts and who have a right to know the information are liable for breach of confidentiality if they share it with others who have no need to know. Those that access patient charts without authorization and no right to know have invaded the patient's privacy. Healthcare workers must vigilantly avoid becoming involved in either situation.

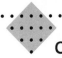

CONCERNS REGARDING COMPUTERIZED PATIENT RECORDS

The goal of preventing inappropriate disclosure of patient information seems overwhelming these days. The explosion of computer technology presents a myriad of challenges to healthcare workers. Most healthcare facilities now maintain at least a partial computerized patient record (CPR) for each patient. In addition, the recent transition from traditional forms of healthcare delivery to the present managed care model has contributed to the challenges of the information age.

"The movement into a managed care environment and the need
for data management systems in healthcare are posing new
legal issues related to maintaining the privacy and confidentiality of
computerized patient records. Many of these concerns are heightened as development continues toward massive patient data-
bases that will be the primary datasystem for numerous networked
managed care providers" [6].

Unfortunately, not all federal and state laws and regulations have
kept pace with the challenges that the CPR presents. In fact, the
federal government just recently proposed standards to address the
security, integrity, confidentiality, and availability of individual
health information pursuant to the Health Insurance Portability and
Accountability Act of 1996 [7].

Health information management professionals and medical assistants, transcriptionists, and secretaries must be thoroughly familiar
with the healthcare provider's data management system and the
pertinent policies and procedures pertaining to it. They must also
have some understanding of the federal and state laws and regulations that affect their job.

SENSITIVE TYPES OF PATIENT INFORMATION

There are four types of patient information that are entitled to
heightened protection from inappropriate disclosure due to the
sensitive nature of the information and the likelihood that it may
form the basis for discrimination (Box 9–2). Patient information that
contains references to the following conditions must be carefully
guarded:

- **Substance abuse**
- **Mental illness**
- **Sexually transmitted diseases**
- **Genetic makeup.**

Genetic makeup has become the latest area to cause concern regarding confidentiality. Scientists have the ability to detect carriers
of certain diseases such as cystic fibrosis, sickle cell anemia, and

---

BOX 9–2 • SENSITIVE PATIENT INFORMATION

Four types of patient information that are entitled to heightened protection from inappropriate disclosure due to the sensitive nature of the information:

1. Substance abuse

2. Mental illness

3. Sexually transmitted diseases

4. Genetic makeup

Huntington's disease. Advances in genetic research and recent collaborations among scientists who are attempting to identify the composition of all human genetic material have greatly enhanced the ability to detect the genes responsible for many more diseases, including various forms of cancer. Some state laws already require special protection of this information [8].

Protection of patient information reflecting a diagnosis with a **sexually transmitted disease** such as HIV and AIDS is clearly required by law because of the social stigma associated with these conditions. Under certain circumstances, some states and the federal government have laws specifically limiting the type and amount of information that can be released from a patient's record. For example, in New Jersey, providers who release information about a patient's **psychological treatment** to a third-party payor, such as a health insurance company, must limit disclosure to administrative information, diagnostic information, patient status, and other general information, providing no specific details regarding sessions and other treatment [9]. At the federal level, specific standards limiting disclosure of medical records containing **substance abuse** information such as drug addiction exist [10]. These are only a few examples of the many state and federal limitations imposed.

MEASURES TO PROTECT THE "CPR"

What are some of the specific measures in place to protect the CPR? Nowadays, each healthcare worker permitted to access the CPR is issued a **confidential personal code (CPC)** or computer password by the employer. The password allows the user a level of access necessary for the user to perform his job. In many states, the regulatory bodies which oversee various healthcare practitioners such as physicians have regulations for maintaining a CPR that specifically address access and use of a CPC and changing CPCs periodically. An example of such a regulation is set forth in Box 9–3. Most employers

---

BOX 9–3 • CPR REGULATIONS

A patient record may be prepared and maintained on a personal or other computer only when it meets the following criteria:

1. The patient record shall contain at least two forms of identification, for example, name and record number or any other specific information.

2. An entry in the patient record shall be made by the physician contemporaneously with the medical service and shall contain the date of service, date of entry, and full printed name of the treatment provider. The physician shall finalize or "sign" the entry by means of a confidential personal code ("CPC") and include date of the "signing."

3. Alternatively, the physician may dictate a dated entry for later transcription. The transcription shall be dated and identified as "preliminary" until reviewed, finalized, and dated by the responsible physician as provided in [2] above.

4. The system shall contain an internal permanently activated date and time recordation for all entries and shall automatically prepare a backup copy of the file.

5. The system shall be designed in such manner that, after "signing" by means of the CPC, the existing entry cannot be changed in any manner. Notwithstanding the permanent status of a prior entry, a new entry may be made at any time and may indicate correction to a prior entry.

6. Where more than one licensee is authorized to make entries into the computer file of any professional treatment record, the physician responsible for the medical practice shall assure that each such person obtains a CPC and uses the file program in the same manner [11].

strictly prohibit the user from sharing the password with anyone else. In fact, employers will discipline an employee who shares the password with others. Disciplinary action may include suspension or possible termination of employment, depending on the facility's policies and the nature of the transgression.

Biometrics

Once the technology becomes more cost effective, more healthcare facilities will begin to utilize **biometrics** in place of passwords to allow healthcare workers access to the CPR. **Biometric identification systems** detect a human physical feature to allow access to computer data. Some examples include fingerprint recognition when an employee touches a special keypad, retina or iris scanning when an employee looks into the computer screen, and voice recognition. This technology will enhance a facility's ability to further restrict inappropriate access to patient information.

Identification

Most CPR systems have the ability to determine the identity of anyone who accesses the system and to detect whether that individual is authorized to do so. CPR systems also have the ability to create audit trails that record all attempts made to access a patient record and all attempts to alter that record. These **audit trails** also detect and trace a breach in security. All healthcare workers should familiarize themselves with their employer's policies and procedures for reporting suspected security breaches of the computer system.

Protection of Information

For the healthcare worker who uses the computer terminal, whether on a regular basis or intermittently, it is important to protect the information from unauthorized viewers. Computer terminals should be positioned so they cannot be seen by those who have no need to view the information. Computer terminals should also utilize an automatic blanking feature so that the screen will go blank if a keystroke is not made within a set period of time. Too often, healthcare workers also leave computer terminals without signing off—a habit that should be avoided so as to prevent an unauthorized user access.

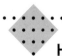

HANDLING REQUESTS AND SUBPOENAS FOR PATIENT RECORDS

Requests for patient records come from a variety of sources including the patient, health insurance carriers, managed care companies, other healthcare providers, and attorneys. All healthcare providers require proper authorization and consent from the patient before such information is released to the requester. Professional groups such as the **Joint Commission on Accreditation of Healthcare Organizations (JCAHO)** mandate such measures. Governmental agencies such as the **Office of the Inspector General (OIG)**, which oversees the prevention and investigation of Medicare and Medicaid fraud and abuse, recommend that facilities adopt compliance programs which address, among other things, policies and procedures for distribution of patient records.

Healthcare facilities frequently receive legal documents such as a subpoena duces tecum. Attorneys often direct such subpoenas to the patient record custodian, commanding the custodian to appear for a deposition and produce a patient's treatment record. State courts and the federal courts have specific rules addressing the proper form, appropriate service, and other requirements necessary for the subpoena to be valid. (See the Federal Rules of Civil Procedure, rule 45, and your state law regarding the subpoena duces tecum.)

In some states, a subpoena duces tecum must state that the documentation requested shall not be produced or released until the date specified for the taking of the deposition. This provision gives opposing counsel, usually the patient's attorney, the opportunity to quash the subpoena. Opposing counsel may have reason to believe that the subpoenaed information is not at issue in the case, is confidential, and should not be released. If that is the case, a motion to quash the subpoena is filed. Therefore, it is important that the medical records custodian not release the documentation sought until the date specified in the subpoena. If the medical records custodian receives oral or written notice that opposing counsel has moved to quash the subpoena or is going to do so, the documentation sought should not be released until the facility is provided with a court order.

If any situation arises in which health information personnel are unsure whether to release patient information in response to a subpoena or other request, the patient (or the patient's attorney if there is one) should be contacted and written authorization obtained.

Special concerns may be raised if the patient record contains any information that is entitled to heightened protection as previously discussed. For example, there may be concerns and uncertainties about releasing medical records containing substance abuse information. Health information personnel should consult the facility's legal counsel before releasing any information if there are concerns or uncertainties as to how to proceed. It is much wiser to exercise caution before the information is released than to attempt to prevent costly litigation after an inappropriate disclosure.

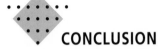

CONCLUSION

Ester Levin (see the case scenario) was rightfully concerned about providing Mr. Farmer with a printout of the healthcare records pertaining to Dr. Lewis. All healthcare information should be considered confidential. Although there are certain exceptions to nondisclosure, none of the exceptions applied. Dr. Lewis did not authorize release of his records, and Mr. Farmer had no need to know what was contained in the healthcare record. In fact, because of possible HIV status, Dr. Lewis' record was entitled to heightened protection.

Although Ms. Levin was afraid that she might be disciplined or fired if she refused to give Mr. Farmer the information he requested, the opposite is true. Had she released the information she would have exposed herself, Mr. Farmer, and the medical center to possible litigation. She may have lost her job as a result of her failure to uphold the medical center's policies regarding nondisclosure. The situation called for Ms. Levin's firm, but polite, refusal to release the information, accompanied by a brief explanation that her department's policies and procedures do not authorize her to comply with his request.

PERTINENT POINTS

1. When in doubt, obtain the patient's consent for release of records.
2. The basic rule of thumb is who has a need to know the information contained in the patient's record.
3. Negligence is different from an intentional tort or quasi-intentional tort.
4. Tort is a civil wrongdoing.

5. Breach of confidentiality is a quasi-intentional tort.
6. Sensitive information includes patient information dealing with:
   a. Genetic makeup
   b. Mental illness
   c. Substance abuse
   d. Sexually transmitted disease.
7. "CPC" means Confidential Personal Code or computer password.
8. Biometric identification systems are developed as an additional security device to protect the release of patient information.
9. A subpoena duces tecum is used to obtain medical records.

STUDY QUESTIONS

1. What does right to privacy mean with regard to healthcare records?

2. What does the need to know exception or rule mean when applied to the release of patient information?

3. Discuss two violations of a patient's right of privacy.

4. Explain how a breach of confidentiality differs from invasion of privacy.

5. What types of patient information are considered sensitive and should receive heightened protection?

6. Describe measures that can be used to protect the patient's computerized record.

7. What is a subpoena duces tecum? How is it commonly used with regard to patient records?

8. Describe to the class situations you have been in or have witnessed that could have resulted in litigation due to an invasion of a patient's privacy or a breach of confidentiality. How could the situation have been handled differently?

9. What is a tort?

10. What is a quasi-intentional tort? Give several examples.

REFERENCES

1. N.J.A.C. 8:43G-15.2 (a) and (b).
2. Aiken, T. (Ed.) (2002). *Legal, ethical and political issues in nursing.* Philadelphia: F.A. Daivs Company.
3. Pierce v. Caday, 244 Va. 285, 422 S.E. 2d 37 (Va., 1992).
4. Estate of *Behringer v. Princeton Medical Center* 592 A.2d 1251, 249 (N.J. Super. 597, 1991).
5. Fairfax Hospital v. Curtis, 492 S.E.2d 642 254 Va. 437 (Va. Super. 1997)
6. Ballard, D. & Cohen, J. W. (1995). Confidentiality of patient records in the computer age. *Journal of Nursing Law* 2(4), 49–61.
7. 63 FR 43242, Proposed Rules, Security and Electronic Signature Standards, August 12, 1998.
8. Scanlon, C. (1998). The legal implications of genetic testing. *RN*, 61–65.
9. N.J.S.A. 45: 14B-32
10. 42 U.S.C. See 290 ee–3
11. N.J.A.C. 13:35-6.5 (3)

10

Clinical Laboratory Liability

DIANE TRACE WARLICK, RN, BSN, JD

▶ Key Chapter Concepts

Negligence
Standards of Care
Practice Guidelines
Clinical Laboratory Improvement
    Amendments
Scope of Duty
Expert Testimony
Spoilation

▶ Objectives

At the conclusion of this chapter, the reader will be able to:

1. Identify the elements of a professional negligence action.

2. Identify at least five sources of standards of care.

3. Discuss the Clinical Laboratory Improvement Amendments.

4. Define "spoilation."

5. Explain the expert testimony requirement and exceptions.

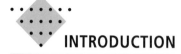

INTRODUCTION

There are many areas of potential legal liability for clinical laboratories, including breach of contract, federal false claims for Medicare and Medicaid billing practices, employer and employee disputes, and negligence. This chapter focuses on areas of potential liability for negligence, also known as malpractice.

▶ Case Scenario

Blood tests were ordered for a patient suffering symptoms of weakness in her lower extremities. The tests were to determine if she had multiple sclerosis or a vitamin B-12 deficiency. The laboratory incorrectly reported a normal range for vitamin B-12 due to an error in methodology. Vitamin B-12 tests were ordered again because the patient's symptoms worsened, but were never done. The patient became permanently paralyzed. Who was liable? What breach of the standards occurred? (This case will be discussed later in the chapter.)

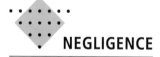

NEGLIGENCE

Negligence is the failure to use such care as a reasonably prudent and careful person would use under similar circumstances; it is the doing of some act which a person of ordinary prudence would not have done under similar circumstances or failure to do what a person of ordinary prudence would have done under similar circumstances[1].

There are four elements to be proven by a claimant, or "plaintiff," in a malpractice action:

1. Duty
2. Breach of duty
3. Causation
4. Damages.

The plaintiff must prove all four elements by a **preponderance of the evidence.** In other words, the jury (or a court sitting as the finder of fact) must determine whether in its collective mind, based upon the evidence presented, it is **more likely than not** that the alleged negligence caused injury to the plaintiff. If so, the jury (or court) will determine the amount by which the plaintiff has been damaged.

STANDARD OF CARE

All persons have a general duty to avoid harming other persons. In the usual negligence case, whether or not a defendant has breached that duty is measured by the **"reasonable person"** standard. In making this determination, the fact finder, jury or judge, must decide whether the defendant has acted as an ordinary reasonable man would have acted under the same or similar circumstances. In **professional negligence actions,** otherwise known as **malpractice actions,** the professional's conduct is measured by the standards of the profession rather than the reasonable person standard. This takes into account the specialized knowledge, skill, and experience of the professional. Professional standards may be embodied in practice guidelines, laws, regulations, or simply the usual day-to-day practices of the members of the profession. These standards must ordinarily be introduced at a trial through the testimony of an expert witness, as discussed below.

One of the early procedural issues to face the courts in malpractice litigation was whether the professional standard against which a defendant's conduct was to be measured was determined by looking solely at the usual practices of members of the profession in the same **locality** as the defendant or **nationally.** At one time, the prevailing rule was that professional conduct was measured against the conduct of other members of the profession meeting the minimum qualifications for licensure in the same or similar locale. **The majority rule now recognizes a national standard of care with respect to medical specialties and other certified or accredited healthcare services, including clinical laboratories.**

The evolution from the local standard and the rationale for a national standard of care in medical negligence cases was directly at issue in *Morrison v. MacNamera* [2].[1] *Morrison* involved a nationally certified clinical laboratory against which a malpractice suit had been

---

[1]The court discussed the issue at great length in a comprehensive review of the case law from across the country on the issue, on both local and national standards of care.

filed by a patient injured during the performance of a urethral smear test. The issue on appeal was whether the laboratory, through its employee, had breached the standard of care by performing the test while the patient was standing. There was an additional issue of whether repeating the test with the patient standing when the patient was feeling faint after the first swab was taken was negligent. Expert witnesses testified for the Washington, D.C., laboratory that it was proper to perform the test with the patient in a standing position and that it was the accepted practice in the locality. Experts from other areas of the country testified to the contrary. The court explained the original reason for the locality standard:

> "This doctrine . . . appears to have developed in the late nine-
> teenth century. . . . The rule was designed to protect doctors in
> rural areas who, because of inadequate training and experience
> and lack of effective means of transportation and communication,
> could not be expected to exhibit the skill and care of urban
> doctors. . . . In sum, the locality rule was premised on the notion
> that the disparity in education and access to advances in
> medical science between rural and urban doctors required that
> they be held to different standards of care."

After a lengthy dissertation on the subject, the court concluded that the standardization of medical education through the country, the availability of medical journals on a nationwide basis, the ubiquitous "detail men" of the drug companies, tape recorded and closed circuit television, medical presentations, hundreds of widely available post-graduate courses, and other factors rendered the locality rule obsolete in medical malpractice cases. The court also noted that simply because everyone in the locality followed a particular procedure did not make a negligent procedure acceptable. The court held that these same reasons apply with equal validity to hold clinical laboratories to a national standard of care.

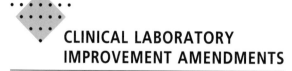

CLINICAL LABORATORY
IMPROVEMENT AMENDMENTS

In *Morrison*, a 1979 case, the laboratory involved was admittedly a national certified clinical laboratory. Today, it would be unusual to find a medical laboratory that is not certified, accredited, or otherwise subject to national regulatory standards. In 1988, Congress passed the **Clinical Laboratory Improvement Amendment** [3].[2] The Clinical Laboratory Improvement Amendment (CLIA) set forth extensive conditions or standards which laboratories[3] must meet to be certified by the U.S. Department of Health and Human Services (HHS).[4] Unless a clinical laboratory is performing only simple, routine tests for which certification has been waived by CLIA,[5] a laboratory must be certified by HHS or another approved accrediting organization to receive payments for services to Medicare or Medicaid beneficiaries. CLIA regulations include standards for proficiency testing by specialty and subspecialty, quality control, quality assurance, personnel qualifications and responsibilities, facilities, equipment, and test specific procedures (Box 10–1). The significance of the regulations to potential malpractice liability is that the comprehensive regulations set a minimum standard against which the conduct of a laboratory or its personnel will be undoubtedly measured in litigation.[6] These standards can be introduced at trial through the testimony of an expert witness as evidence of the laboratory's breach of duty of care to its clients. If the failure of the laboratory to meet these regulatory standards causes injury to a patient, malpractice liability will be difficult to avoid.[7]

---

[2]It should be noted that as of January 2000, the states of Washington and New York were exempt from CLIA regulations. In nonexempt states, there were 175 clinical laboratories certified under CLIA, of which 58% were privately operated (www.hfca.gov/medicaid/clia/statupda.htm).

[3]Laboratory is defined as "a facility for the biological, microbiological, serological, chemical, immunohematological, hematological, biophysical, cytological, pathological or other examination of materials derived from the human body for the purpose of providing information for the diagnosis, prevention, or treatment of any disease or impairment of, or the assessment of the health of human beings . . ." 42 C.F.R. 493.2.

[4]The regulations implementing CLIA are codified at 42 Code of Federal Regulations, Part 493. They can be found on the internet at www.phppo.cdc.gov/dis/clia/docs/42cfr49399.htm.

[5]A list of waived tests is set forth in the regulations at 42 C.F.R. 493.15.

[6]The unexcused violation of a statute or regulation enacted for the safety of the public that is applicable under the circumstances is *per se* or automatic negligence in some states. This rule is known as "**negligence per se**" states, proof of "violation" of the safety statute or regulation establishes the breach of duty.

[7]Although the overall burden of proof on a plaintiff in a negligence action is "**preponderance of the evidence**" or "**more likely than not**," an expert's testimony with respect to the cause of the plaintiff's injury must meet a more stringent standard in most jurisdictions. The expert must testify that the breach of the standard of care probably, not possibly, caused the injury (e.g., *Denneny v. Siegal,* 407 F.2d 433, 400-41 (3rd Cir. 1969).

BOX 10–1 • CLIA QUALITY CONTROL FOR TESTS OF MODERATE COMPLEXITY, HIGH COMPLEXITY, OR ANY COMBINATION OF THESE TESTS

This part of the Code of Federal Regulations (42 C.F.R. Part 493, Subpart K) includes standards and conditions for the following:

- 493.1203 Standard: Moderate- or high-complexity testing, or both, effective December 31, 2000.
- 493.1204 Standard: Facilities.
- 493.1204 Standard: Test methods, equipment, instrumentation, reagents, materials, and supplies.
- 493.1211 Standard: Procedure manual.
- 493.1213 Standard: Establishment and verification of method performance.
- 493.1215 Standard: Equipment maintenance and function checks.
- 493.1217 Standard: Calibration and calibration verification procedures.
- 493.1218 Standard: Control procedures.
- 493.1219 Standard: Remedial actions.
- 493.1221 Standard: Quality control records.
- 493.1223 Standard: Condition: Quality control—specialties and subspecialties for tests of moderate and high complexity.
- 493.1225 Condition: Microbiology.
- 493.1227 Condition: Bacteriology.
- 493.1229 Condition: Microbacteriology.
- 493.1231 Condition: Mycology.
- 493.1233 Condition: Parasitology.
- 493.1235 Condition: Virology.
- 493.1237 Condition: Diagnostic immunology.
- 493.1239 Condition: Syphillis serology.
- 493.1241 Condition: General immunology.
- 493.1243 Condition: Chemistry.
- 493.1245 Condition: Routine chemistry.
- 493.1247 Condition: Endocrinology.

Box continued on opposite page

**BOX 10–1 • CLIA QUALITY CONTROL FOR TESTS
OF MODERATE COMPLEXITY, HIGH COMPLEXITY,
OR ANY COMBINATION OF THESE TESTS** *CONTINUED*

- 493.1249 Condition: Toxicology.

- 493.1251 Condition: Urinalysis.

- 493.1255 Condition: Pathology.

- 493.1259 Condition: Histopathology.

- 493.1261 Condition: Oral pathology.

- 493.1263 Condition: Radiobioassay.

- 493.1265 Condition: Histocompatibility.

- 493.1267 Condition: Clinical cytogenics.

- 493.1269 Condition: Immunohematology.

- 493.1271 Condition: Transfusion services and blood banking.

- 493.1273 Standard: Immunohematological collection, processing, dating periods, labeling, and distribution of blood and blood products.

- 493.1275 Standard: Blood and blood product storage facilities.

- 493.1277 Standard: Arrangement for services.

- 493.1283 Standard: Provision of testing.

- 493.1283 Standard: Retention of samples of transfused blood.

- 493.1285 Standard: Investigation of transfusion reactions.

SOURCES OF STANDARDS

Additional federal regulations apply to clinical laboratories located in hospital facilities. The **Conditions of Participation for Hospitals for Laboratory Services** [4] specifically incorporate all CLIA standards and make them applicable to hospital facilities. Other regulations applicable to hospital laboratories are included, which are principally directed toward handling of potentially infected blood and blood products. Professional organizations also promulgate standards and guidelines that may be introduced at trial to establish a duty and prove breach of that duty in a laboratory malpractice action. The American Board of Clinical Chemistry[8] offers certification in clinical chemistry, toxicological chemistry, and molecular diagnostics to individuals with doctoral level degrees. The board establishes standards of competence for those who practice clinical laboratory medicine (www.aacc.org/abcc/). The American Association for Clinical Chemistry (same address as the American Board of Clinical Chemistry, footnote 8) maintains a list of standard materials and standard methods compiling the most up-to-date information on clinical laboratory standardization available to its Standards Committee.[9] The National Academy of Clinical Biochemistry publishes "Laboratory Medicine Practice Guidelines" (LMPG) for the application of clinical biochemistry to medical diagnosis and therapy. Standards may also be established by a laboratory's own **internal policies and procedures** manuals.

EXPERT TESTIMONY

Expert testimony is generally required to establish the applicable standard of care in laboratory malpractice actions as in other medical malpractice cases. The testimony of an expert[10] in clinical laboratory science or other related disciplines is necessary to explain the technical and scientific data needed by a jury of lay persons to identify the appropriate standard of care and determine whether that standard has been breached. One exception to the expert testimony requirement, known as the **"common knowledge" exception,** was at issue in *Schindel v. Albany Medical Corporation* [5]. **This exception applies where "the defendant's negligence is so grossly apparent or the treatment is so common that a lay person can readily appraise it using his everyday knowledge"** [6].

---

[8]ABCC, 2101 L Street, N.W., Suite 202, Washington, DC 20037-1526 (phone 202-835-8727; fax 202-887-5039).

[9]Standards are available on line at www.aacc.org/standards/analyses.stm.

[10]An individual may qualify to testify as an expert in litigation based upon his or her knowledge, skill, experience, training, or education in the field. It is the function of the trial judge as a "gatekeeper" to determine whether an individual qualifies to testify as an expert. Rule 702, Federal Rules of Evidence; *U.S. v. Webb,* 115 F.3d 711 (9th Cir. 1997); *Wood v. Minnesota Mining and Manufacturing Co.,* 112 F.3d 306, 309 (8th Cir. 1997); *Bogosian v. Mercedes-Benz,* 104 F.3d 472, 476 (1st Cir. 1997).

In *Schindel,* a woman sought an abortion at a local women's clinic. The laboratory analysis of the tissue following the procedure indicated the possibility of an ectopic pregnancy that was not terminated by the abortion procedure. The testimony at trial established that while the physician had a duty to review the laboratory report to identify any abnormal results, it was the duty of the laboratory personnel to notify the patient of the findings and give her instructions. In *Schindel,* alleged efforts to notify the plaintiff by mail and telephone were unsuccessful, the plaintiff did not receive notice, and the ectopic pregnancy ruptured. The plaintiff alleged that the defendant was negligent in failing to employ and enforce proper procedures to notify her of the abnormal laboratory findings and failed to notify her of the possible ectopic pregnancy. Without expert testimony to establish the standard of care, the jury returned a verdict for the plaintiff.

On appeal, the laboratory successfully argued that the verdict should be reversed owing to the lack of expert testimony. The court found that the common knowledge exception did not apply to the case even though neither the quality of treatment nor the correctness of the physician's diagnosis was at issue. The court concluded that it was the "urgency of the danger involved and the likelihood and extent of harm to the plaintiff which would dictate the extent of the defendant's duty to notify the plaintiff," and these factors required expert testimony.

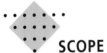

SCOPE OF DUTY

Another aspect of the legal concept of duty in a malpractice case is whether a duty to a particular individual exists under the circumstances. In the physician-patient context, a physician's duty to provide medical care that meets accepted minimum standards attached at the inception of the physician-patient relationship. As in the physician context, the contours and scope of a laboratory's duty of care are not always a bright line. **In a recent Wyoming Supreme Court case [7], the question was whether there was a duty owed by a specimen collection company to an employee of the employer which had hired the company to collect urine specimens for drug and alcohol screening.** The Supreme Court of Wyoming held that there was a duty, overruling the lower court. To collect urine specimens from randomly selected employees, the employer had retained the collection company. The collection company contracted with another laboratory to analyze the specimens and report the results. The plaintiff was randomly selected for testing, gave a specimen in an unsealed container, and then returned to the restroom to wash his hands. In his absence, the container was sealed and the plaintiff was directed to initial the label. Plaintiff's employer was subsequently notified that the laboratory results demonstrated a 0.32 urine alcohol content, which indicated the plaintiff would have been **grossly drunk** at the time of his testing, 10 hours into his shift. Based on this report, the plaintiff was terminated from his employment. The plaintiff filed suit against the collection company alleging that the employee who collected the specimen:

1. Was inadequately trained;
2. Failed to employ proper procedures;
3. Failed to inform the plaintiff that urinalysis specific procedures were not followed; and
4. Misrepresented to the plaintiff the accuracy and reliability of urine alcohol testing.

The court explained that a duty exists where, "upon the facts in evidence, such a relation exists between the parties that the community will impose a legal obligation upon one for the benefit of the other—or more simply, whether the interest of the plaintiff which has suffered invasion was entitled to legal protection at the hands of the defendant" [8]. The court noted that other courts were in disagreement with its opinion on the issue.[11]

Determination of the existence of a duty, according to the Wyoming Supreme Court, requires balancing of the following:

1. **The foreseeability of harm to the plaintiff;**
2. **The closeness of the connection between the defendant's conduct and the injury suffered;**
3. **The degree of certainty that the plaintiff suffered injury;**
4. **The moral blame attached to the defendant's conduct;**
5. **The policy of preventing future harm;**

---

[11]See *Smithkline Beecham Corp. v. Doe*, 903 S.W.2d 347 (Tex. 1995), and *Willis v. Roche Biomedical Labs, Inc.*, 61 F.3d 313, 316 (5th Cir. 1995) finding that a drug tester retained by an employer to screen potential employees owes no duty to that potential employee. See also *Caputo v. Compuchem Laboratories*, Civ.A. No. 92-6123, 1994 WL 100084 (E.D.Pa., Feb. 23, 1994), and *Herbert v. Placid Refining Co.*, 564 So.2d 371, 374 (La.App.), writ denied, 569 So.2d 981 (La. 1990).

6. The extent of the burden upon the defendant;

7. The consequences to the community and the court system; and

8. The availability, cost, and prevalence of insurance for the risk involved.

In the recent case *Santos v. Kim* [9], the existence of a duty owed by the director of a medical laboratory and the plaintiff mother of a deceased newborn was discussed at length. **The question was whether the director was potentially liable for the laboratory's failure to have policies and procedures in place for assuring that treating physicians were promptly notified of abnormal test results.** The court noted that in modern medical practice, it was not always necessary that there be a personal relationship or actual physical contact between the healthcare provider and patient because in many instances it is the technician with the least knowledge and skill who actually interacts directly with the patient, as often occurs in radiology and laboratory services. Mrs. Santos was Rh negative, and this was her second pregnancy. Her obstetricians had been monitoring her anti-D titers on a biweekly basis to assure prompt treatment of Rh incompatibility, if necessary. The week the titers rose substantially, the obstetricians were not notified of the abnormal result for 2 weeks. In the meantime, Mrs. Santos underwent a Cesarean section without prophylactic treatment, which allegedly led to the death of the neonate. **The Massachusetts Supreme Court held that under this set of circumstances, the medical director of the laboratory could potentially be liable to Mrs. Santos even though he had no direct contact with her at any time.**

COMMON AREAS OF LABORATORY LIABILITY

Common sources of professional liability (Box 10–2) for clinical laboratories based upon reported malpractice cases include the following:

- Error in diagnostic testing for cancer
- False positive drug screening reported to employers
- Unidentified tainted blood products
- Failure to identify genetic disorders in newborns and pregnancy screening

- Delay in or failure to transmit laboratory results
- Use of improper equipment or procedures.

In most reported court cases, whether or not there was negligent conduct by the defendant(s) is not the issue before the court. The court opinions discuss various procedural questions in the context of the malpractice action in which the inappropriateness of the conduct is not questioned. (Most cases which do not have unresolved legal issues to be decided are ultimately settled by the parties and therefore not reported in the case law.)

Pathology errors are very common sources of malpractice liability for clinical laboratories, with allegedly misread Pap smears heading the list. In none of the cases reviewed was the negligence of the conduct even discussed. In *Calvin v. Schlossman* [10], the issue was whether an action alleging the laboratory was culpable for an error in reading a Pap smear is subject to state law prelitigation hearing procedures applicable to medical malpractice actions. The court held that it was. In *Riseman v. Goldberg* [11], the question was whether it was the private physician who ordered a test or the hospital which operated the laboratory that was vicariously responsible for the pathologist's error in reading a Pap smear specimen.[12] In *Berg v.*

---

[12]**Vicarious liability** is defined as indirect legal responsibility, for example, the liability of an employer for the acts of an employee, or a principal for the torts and contracts of an agent. *Black's Law Dictionary* (5th ed., West, 1971).

BOX 10–2 • COMMON AREAS OF LABORATORY LIABILITY

- Errors in reading Pap smears
- False positive drug screening reported to employers
- Unidentified tainted blood products
- Failure to identify genetic disorders in newborns and pregnancy screening
- Delay in or failure to transmit laboratory results
- Use of improper equipment or procedures

Footer [12], liability to the plaintiff was stipulated. The only question was whether the settling defendant was a "joint tortfeasor" for purposes of determining the allowable deduction from the judgment owed plaintiff by the nonsettling defendant. *Bergherr v. Sommer* [13] discusses whether a Minnesota court has jurisdiction over an out-of-state laboratory in which specimens were "off-loaded" by a laboratory in Minnesota. The court ruled it had jurisdiction because the out-of-state laboratory actively solicited business from Minnesota through its agreements with the Minnesota laboratory and benefited economically from "voluntary interstate economic activity."

Marsh v. Wentzel [14] deals with the statute of limitations for misdiagnosed breast cancer which was not discovered until after the 4-year time limit for bringing suit had expired. *Henry v. Metropolitan Government of Nashville* [15] points out that even though there may be negligent conduct, if the negligence does not cause any damage, there is no basis to recover in a malpractice lawsuit and the case will be dismissed. Ms. Henry had a Pap smear in July 1993 which was positive for cervical cancer, but she was never informed of the results. In October 1994, she had another Pap smear that was reported to her as positive, and as a result she had surgery. The testimony of experts established that although there was a 14-month delay in notifying her of the cervical cancer, there was no damage because she underwent the same surgery she would have had earlier had the diagnosis been made earlier. Accordingly, there was no harm suffered and the case was dismissed.

Equipment and procedural errors are often the subject of laboratory liability cases. In *National Health Laboratories v. Pari* [16], an error in testing methodology resulted in a $10 million verdict for a patient permanently paralyzed owing to an error in diagnosis. Blood tests were ordered for the plaintiff suffering symptoms of weakness in her lower extremities, to differentiate between possible multiple sclerosis or vitamin B-12 deficiency. The laboratory admitted the error in methodology, based upon which the technicians incorrectly reached a normal range finding for vitamin B-12. When the symptoms worsened, the patient was admitted to the hospital and vitamin B-12 tests were again ordered, but this time the order was never carried out. The laboratory and the hospital were both held to be 50% responsible for the plaintiff's resulting paralysis and damages.

AIDS- and hepatitis-tainted blood products were areas of significant liability for laboratories and hospitals in the early 1980s before AIDS was identified and a reliable test existed to screen blood products for HIV contamination, even in the absence of negligence. Many states now have statutes that preclude strict liability or liability without fault in these cases,[13] although liability for negligent screening still exists. In *Smith v. County of Kern* [17], a laboratory performed the wrong test on a blood sample. An HIV test was ordered pursuant to state law for the benefit of a police officer exposed to the blood of a patient who said he tried to commit suicide because he suffered from AIDS. The blood sample given by this patient was erroneously tested for hepatitis instead of the HIV virus, but the remaining sample was discarded before the error was discovered. The patient had also been discharged, leaving no forwarding address by this time. It took over 6 months to locate the patient to obtain another sample and perform the proper tests. The court agreed there was possible liability for the 6-month delay in obtaining results of the HIV test.

While "spoilation" was not an issue in the *Smith* case, the **spoilation doctrine** has been developing over the last decade as both an evidentiary rule and a source of punishment or of "sanctions" against defendants and their attorneys who lose or destroy evidence or alter records. **Spoilation is defined as the intentional destruction of evidence which, when established, allows the court to instruct the jury that it may infer that the lost or damaged evidence was unfavorable to the party responsible for the spoilation** [18]. It includes "the destruction or the significant and meaningful alteration of a document or instrument." In *Aldrich v. Roche Biomedical Laboratories, Inc.* [19], the court concluded there was no spoilation because it could not be definitively determined how the pathology slides disappeared or by whom. The pathology slides that were questionably misread disappeared in the court or after being returned by mail from an expert reviewing the slides for a second opinion. The loss of the slides was ultimately determined not to impact the presentation of the case.

The Clinical Laboratory Improvement Amendments contain specific requirements for recordkeeping and preservation of samples. Records of patient testing, including printed results, must be kept for at least 2 years [20]. Immunohematology records, transfusion records, and records of blood and blood product testing must be retained at least 5 years. Therefore, not only does the laboratory have a duty not to lose, alter, or destroy records, it has an affirmative duty to maintain them.

---

[13]For example, Pennsylvania Blood Shield Statute, more specifically titled "Body Fluid and Tissue Limited Civil Immunity Act," 42 Pa.C.S.A. subsection 8333 (1982 and Supp. 2000); Missouri Blood Shield Statute, subsection 431.069 R.S. Mo. 1978.

BOX 10–3 • LABORATORY ACCREDITING ORGANIZATIONS APPROVED BY HCFA

- Commission on Office Laboratory Accreditation
- College of American Pathologists
- Joint Commission on Accreditation of Health Care Organizations
- American Osteopathic Association
- American Association of Blood Banks
- American Society of Histocompatibility and Immunogenics

Source: CLIA Update, Division of Laboratories and Acute Care Services, Health Care Financing Administration, January, 2000. www.hcfa.gov/medicaid/clia/statuada.htm

---

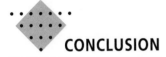

CONCLUSION

As in other areas of healthcare liability, theories of liability evolve as professional standards change. It is incumbent upon the practitioner to constantly stay abreast of new standards and regulations, to be familiar with and follow in-house policies and procedures, and to question out-of-date practices, equipment, and methodologies (Box 10–3).

STUDY QUESTIONS

1. What are the elements of negligence?

2. List four areas of potential legal liability for clinical laboratories.

3. Discuss local versus national standards of care. How do they differ?

4. Find a case in your field at the law library or on-line and discuss the elements of negligence.

5. What are the Clinical Laboratory Improvement Amendments?

6. List three sources of standards for your area of practice.

7. List six common areas of laboratory liability and how to prevent lawsuits in each area.

8. Find and discuss a case in the following areas:

   a. Pathology error

   b. Misdiagnosed cancer

   c. Equipment error

   d. Procedural error

   e. AIDS-tainted blood products

   f. Hepatitis-tainted blood products.

9. What is spoilation of evidence?

10. What is the burden of proof on a plaintiff in a negligence action?

REFERENCES

1. *Black's law dictionary* (5th ed.) (1971) (p. 930). St. Paul, MN: West.
2. Morrison v. MacNamera, 407 A.2d 555 (D.C.App. 1979).
3. Clinical Laboratory Improvement Amendment, P.L. 100-578.
4. Conditions of Participation for Hospitals for Laboratory Services, 42 C.F.R. 482.27.
5. Schindel v. Albany Medical Corporation, 625 N.E.2d 114, 252 Ill.App.3d 389 (Ill. App. 1993).
6. Id. at 119.
7. Duncan v. Afton, Inc., 991 P.2d 739 (Wyo. 1999).
8. *Prosser and Keeton on torts* (5th ed.) (1984) (p. 236). St. Paul, MN: West.
9. Santos v. Kim, 706 N.E.2d 658 (Mass. 1999).
10. Calvin v. Schlossman, 427 N.Y.S.2d 632, 74 A.D. 265 (N.Y.App.Div. 1980).
11. Riseman v. Goldberg, 581 N.Y.S.2d 854, 181 A.D. 873 (N.Y.App.Div. 1992).
12. Berg v. Footer, 673 A.2d 1244 (D.C. 1996).
13. Bergherr v. Sommer, 523 N.W.2d 17 (Minn.App. 1994).
14. Marsh v. Wentzel, 732 So.2d 985 (Ala. 1998).
15. Henry v. Metropolitan Government of Nashville, App. Lexis 303 (Tenn. 1999).
16. National Health Laboratories v. Pari, 596 A.2d 555 (D.C. 1991).
17. Smith v. County of Kern, 20 Cal.App.4th 1826, 25 Cal.Rptr.2d 716 (Cal.App.Dist. 5 1993).
18. *Black's law dictionary* (6th ed.) (1990) (p. 1401). St. Paul, MN: West.
19. Aldrich v. Roche Biomedical Laboratories, Inc., 737 So.2d 1124 (Fla. App. Dist. 5 1999).
20. 42 C.F.R. 493.1107, Standard: Test records.

11

Medical Equipment Liability and Litigation

JAN SIMONEAUX, RN, MN

▶ Objectives

At the conclusion of this chapter, the reader should be able to:

1. Define the liability that arises in professions when using medical equipment.

2. Identify potential and/or actual medical equipment litigation.

3. Discuss the Safe Medical Device Act of 1990.

4. Discuss common areas of liability for licensed professionals.

5. Identify strategies for reducing and/or eliminating liability.

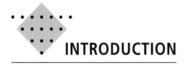

INTRODUCTION

The focus of this chapter is addressing common areas of liability and litigation associated with medical equipment. The chapter provides information related to medical equipment liability and litigation, examples of medical equipment liability and litigation, and strategies for reducing and/or eliminating liability associated with use of medical equipment.

▶ Case Scenario

In an effort to alleviate a stricture, a patient had a Foley catheter inserted during surgery. Several days later, healthcare providers discovered a tiny hole in the balloon of the catheter that allowed urine to leak through to the suture line and into the tissue. This situation caused the patient to undergo two additional surgeries. Who was found negligent? Why? What would you do if you are named in a lawsuit for being negligent in providing safe care to a client? You pride yourself as being a very competent and knowledgeable professional. As you investigate the situation, you learn that the negligence is related to a malfunctioning piece of equipment. You are puzzled because you reported that piece of faulty equipment to your supervisor. What can you do? What should you have done? How could you have prevented the injury to the patient?

Liability is an individual's responsibility for his conduct for failure to meet a standard of care or for failure to perform a duty that causes harm to a client [1,2]. **Strict liability** differs in that liability may be proven without demonstrating fault. **Product liability** is related to liability of a manufacturer or vendor for injury to a person by a given product [2].

Is the issue of liability the equipment or the operator? What do you think as you read the following?

- *A burn is caused from a heating pad placed on a shivering infant* [3].
- *A patient is left without oxygen for a period of time while a caregiver looks for a portable tank* [4].
- *Medication burn occurs to a patient's chest wall incision from Nipride leaking through a pinhole in an atrial catheter during surgery* [5].
- *Equipment is substituted because the right equipment is not available* [6].

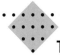

THE SAFE MEDICAL DEVICE ACT OF 1990 (SMDA)

What constitutes a medical device or medical equipment? A **medical device** is a broad term encompassing such items as implants, single use of disposable devices, instruments, machines, apparatus, and reagents. **The Safe Medical Devices Act of 1990 (SMDA)** provides rules and regulations for the safety and reporting of medical devices. As of July 31, 1996, the SMDA requires reporting of incidents [7]. **Sentinel events** are voluntarily reported to the Joint Commission on the Accreditation of Hospitals. This may become mandatory in the near future. If an organization is to provide information that reasonably suggests that a device or piece of equipment may have contributed to a patient's death, then the organization must file a report with the Food and Drug Administration and manufacturer of the device within 10 days. With a serious injury suspicion, the organization must report to the manufacturer of the device [7,8].

As technology advances and healthcare continues to be complex, liability risk may increase. The risk does not increase for an organization alone. Individuals assume equal risk and professional responsibility to assure knowledge and competency of those advances. Medical equipment has incorporated the use of computerization or information systems technology. For many individuals who are still not comfortable with computerization, this technology poses a new challenge. Identifying one's need for knowledge and education, assuming responsibility for obtaining that education, and assuring competency through mentorship and certifications are safeguards to potential liabilities for the healthcare professional and organization.

Registered nurses and licensed allied healthcare professionals (such as physical therapists, occupational therapists, and respiratory therapists) take an oath to safeguard the client through competent and responsible actions. Professional associations have established codes of ethics that are utilized to uphold the standards of practice. Though each profession has its own uniqueness, many of the standards are similar:

- *Respecting human dignity [9–12].*
- *Safeguarding the client's right to privacy and maintaining confidentiality [9–12].*
- *Providing safe and competent care to clients [9–12].*
- *Maintaining professional competence and participate in activities to further develop one's education and body of knowledge [9–12].*
- *Safeguarding the client/public from misinformation [9–12].*
- *Collaborating with other healthcare professionals to promote efforts to meet the needs of the community or client [9–12].*

WHO IS LIABLE IN EQUIPMENT CASES?

Cases of malpractice and negligence tend to revolve around practice issues such as **medication errors, treatment errors,** and **surgical errors. Medical equipment liability** continues to grow in the number of lawsuits, especially in the era of advanced technology and the increased use of healthcare devices and equipment. Injury from a device or medical equipment may involve a primary caregiver, organization, and/or equipment manufacturer [13].

Negligence theory or **product liability** law may be applied to medical equipment liability. **Product liability** is different from malpractice in that the patient may not have to prove a deviation from a standard of care if the courts apply a strict liability standard. With a strict liability standard, the equipment's manufacturer may be held liable. However, this is not enough; manufacturers may defend by claiming the negligence to be **"user error"** [13] (Case Example 11–1).

▶ Case Example 11–1

A patient is on intravenous (IV) Heparin at an ordered rate of 10 cc per hour. Upon checking the IV, a nurse discovers the pump set for 110 cc per hour, 11 times the prescribed dose. The patient's clotting time is at a potentially dangerous level. The patient expired[14]. Certainly, this is a gross medication error. Is this a medical equipment error as well? No, the error that occurred was a "user error" of the equipment.

MEDICATION ADMINISTRATION

Is medication administration competency really any different from user or operator competency? Medication administration requires knowledge of the medication, indication, side effects, adverse reactions, dosage, administration, and outcome. It is a professional's responsibility to know and understand medication prior to administration of the medication. Medical equipment requires knowledge of the equipment, indication for use, troubleshooting, resource management, and outcome.

COMMON TYPES OF ERRORS

Most errors or liabilities occur from lack of knowledge, failure to communicate, failure to follow through, failure to document, misuse, or carelessness [1] (see Box 11–1). In the case of a 5-month-old boy who was shivering postoperatively, a heating pad was placed on the infant to warm him. The infant sustained second- and third-degree burns to his buttocks, discovered upon assessment [3]. In the case of transferring a patient to a new room, the oxygen flow meter did not secure in the outlet; the caregiver proceeded to find an oxygen tank leaving the patient without oxygen. The patient went into respiratory arrest and expired [4]. Equipment that is malfunctioning must be taken out of service. Also, continued assessment and evaluation of patient care is an absolute to assure meeting the standards of care.

BOX 11–1 • REASONS FOR ERROR

1. Lack of knowledge
2. Failure to communicate
3. Failure to follow through
4. Failure to document
5. Misuse
6. Carelessness

STRATEGIES FOR REDUCING OR ELIMINATING LIABILITIES

Perioperative nursing has published numerous articles on electrosurgical safety and measures to maintain safety in the perioperative setting. The American Association of Operating Room Nurses Recommended Practices Committee (1998) developed five recommended practice strategies as follows:

1. Products are to be safe, meet the needs identified, and promote quality patient care.
2. A mechanism for evaluation and standardization of medical equipment should be implemented.
3. Evaluation of products should be based on objective criteria specific to the function and use of the device.
4. A trial evaluation should be conducted and analyzed.
5. Written policies and procedures must be readily available.

Other strategies to reduce and/or eliminate medical equipment liability and litigation include the following:

- *Increase in knowledge of the equipment*—learn its purpose and indication for use

- *User competency*—obtain training specific to the equipment and troubleshooting strategies
- *Communication*—maintain clear and concise communication with all personnel
- *Follow through*—ensure that faulty equipment is taken out of service and labeled, document out of service, and obtain working equipment for the patient's needs
- *Documentation*—ensure that proper documentation is reflected in the medical record; concerns may be documented on a quality report; medical equipment failure should be reported according to rules and regulations
- *Misuse and/or carelessness*—address with colleagues and with management team.

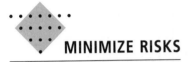

MINIMIZE RISKS

For all licensed healthcare professionals, practice must continuously be monitored. Individual responsibility for continuing education and keeping up to date is of the utmost importance. Areas in which healthcare professionals must invest their time include new technologies, new treatment modalities, equipment advances, medications, and policies/procedures. (See Box 11–2 for common medical equipment encountered in various health professions.) Healthcare professionals must also be familiar with their respective code of ethics, professional standards, and accreditation standards [15].

Competence is the ability to provide a level of care according to a standard of care and according to the profession's code of ethics. **Incompetence** is the failing of moral commitment in upholding the code of ethics. Incompetence jeopardizes patient safety and well-being. Furthermore, colleagues are placed at risk when unable to depend on their team member [10,16].

Why does incompetence occur? Apathy, inability to do the work, disorganization, lack or knowledge of necessary pathophysiology, lack of manual dexterity, or irresponsibility are several reasons for incompetence. Incompetence is generally easily recognizable, yet allowed or tolerated. Haddad [16] points out three reasons for seemingly tolerating incompetence, as follows:

Text continued on page 200

BOX 11–2 • COMMON MEDICAL EQUIPMENT THAT HEALTHCARE PROFESSIONALS MAY ENCOUNTER

Nursing Assistants/Medical Assistants

1. Blood pressure monitors
2. Cardiac monitors
3. Heart catheters
4. Foley catheters
5. Heat lamps
6. Wheelchairs
7. Compression stockings
8. Chest tubes
9. Gomco

Respiratory

1. Ventilators
2. Oxygen flow meters
3. Respiratory treatments
4. Pulse oximetry
5. Compressed air meters
6. Pulmonary function

Physical Therapy

1. Wound care
2. Whirlpool
3. Exercise equipment
4. Ambulation belts
5. Walkers, canes
6. Pulsevac system
7. Continuous positive motion (CPM) machine

Box continued on opposite page

BOX 11–2 • COMMON MEDICAL EQUIPMENT THAT HEALTHCARE PROFESSIONALS MAY ENCOUNTER
Continued

Dental Assistants/Hygienists

1. X-ray machine
2. Ultrasonic scaler/sonic scaler
3. Airbrasive unit
4. Air polisher
5. Slow-speed handpiece/high-speed handpiece
6. Dental unit
7. Ultrasonic unit
8. Autoclave/chemclave machine
9. X-ray developer
10. Automated periodontal probe
11. Computer—chairside and front office
12. Intraoral camera
13. Amalgam tritrator
14. Curing light
15. Model trimmer
16. Stone or plaster
17. Vacuum former
18. Power mixing machine
19. Lathe
20. Panorex machine
21. Pulp vitality tester
22. Nitrous oxide unit
23. Automated irrigating syringe
24. Electrocautery machine
25. Apex locator
26. Casting machine

Box continued on following page

BOX 11–2 • COMMON MEDICAL EQUIPMENT THAT HEALTHCARE PROFESSIONALS MAY ENCOUNTER
Continued

Occupational Therapy

1. Stoves
2. Washing machines
3. Games

Nursing

1. Electronic thermometers
2. Blood pressure cuff with sphygmomanometer
3. Stethoscope
4. Intravenous pumps
5. Emerson or Gomco units
6. Tube feeding pumps
7. Aqua heating pads (e.g., K pads)
8. Hypothermia unit
9. Telemetry transmitters and monitors
10. Bedside electrocardiogram monitors
11. Balloon pumps
12. Cardiac monitor and defibrillator
13. Variety of specialty beds, such as low air loss, rotation beds, fluidized air beds
14. Wheelchair stretchers
15. Walkers
16. Blood glucose meters
17. Automatic external defibrillator

Box continued on opposite page

BOX 11–2 • COMMON MEDICAL EQUIPMENT THAT HEALTHCARE PROFESSIONALS MAY ENCOUNTER
Continued

Cardiology

1. Electrocardiographic unit and leads
2. Treadmill
3. Cardiac ultrasound unit
4. ECG or EKG

Laboratory

1. Hematology and chemistry equipment

Perioperative Services (SDS/OR/PACU)

1. Electrocautery unit
2. Operating room tables
3. Operating room instruments
4. Anesthesia machine that includes oxygen and nitrous oxide sources

Radiology

1. General x-ray or radiographic unit, stationary or mobile
2. Fluoroscopy unit
3. Nuclear medicine unit
4. Magnetic resonance imaging
5. Computed tomography
6. Digital radiography
7. Mammography
8. Lithotriptors
9. Laser
10. Angiography or cardiac catheterization equipment
11. Lead apron
12. Stretchers

Box continued on following page

BOX 11–2 • COMMON MEDICAL EQUIPMENT THAT HEALTHCARE PROFESSIONALS MAY ENCOUNTER *Continued*

Ultrasound

1. Ultrasound Doppler
2. Ultrasound unit
3. Ultrasound scanners
4. Ultrasound transducers

---

1. Loyalty to colleagues—based on a nature to trust, allowances will be made for a person's shortcomings.
2. Principle of beneficence—do good for others.
3. The ability of the incompetent professional to manipulate colleagues—place blame.

Competence equals professionalism; therefore, incompetence cannot be tolerated. It is the responsibility of all professionals to maintain standards and to report a deviation in those standards. Loyalty and beneficence cannot be allowed to blur reality. Patient and colleague safety is at stake.

Continued competency is now required in most states and for most professions. A variety of mechanisms are utilized to determine continued competency, such as self-evaluations, continuing education programs, and peer review. Mandatory continuing education is required by most state boards. The cost associated with continuing education is substantial; effectiveness of such education is not as easy to document [17]. Investment in training and continuing education minimizes the areas of clinical negligence [18].

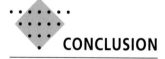

CONCLUSION

In our case scenario discussed at the beginning of the chapter, the hospital was found negligent because the Foley catheter had not been tested prior to insertion. The standard of care is to test the catheter balloon prior to insertion. This standard of care was introduced as evidence against the hospital [19].

Medical equipment liability poses a new challenge in an advanced technological world. Not only has equipment advanced, so has treatment modalities, medications, and standards advanced. Liabilities are much greater. Knowledge, communication, and competency are key components to reducing and eliminating liabilities. Competency is the key to survival and the heart of one's profession.

PERTINENT POINTS

1. Liability is an individual's or organization's responsibility to meet the standard of care for the respective practice or profession.

2. The Safe Medical Devices Act of 1990 provides rules and regulations for safety of equipment and the reporting of serious injuries and/or deaths related to malfunctioning equipment.

3. Technological advances and complex health care will continue to be challenges for all professions.

4. Professional codes of ethics are safeguards for professional practice.

5. Continued competency must be monitored. Incompetence must not be tolerated.

6. Competence equals professionalism.

7. Failure to communicate, failure to follow through, and failure to document are three key areas when liability occurs.

8. Knowledge, communication, and competency are key components to reducing and/or eliminating liabilities.

STUDY QUESTIONS

1. Differentiate liability, strict liability, and product liability.

2. What constitutes a medical device or medical equipment?

3. What does SMDA mean?

4. Name at least three codes of ethics that are similar among the American Association of Respiratory Care, American Physical Therapy Association, and the American Occupational Therapists Association or your profession.

5. What should a caregiver do when incompetence has been identified?

6. What are common areas of medical equipment liability?

7. Identify at least five strategies for reducing and/or eliminating liabilities related to medical equipment.

8. What are common thread "failures" to medical equipment liabilities as well as other liabilities?

REFERENCES

1. Aiken, T. D., & Catalano, J. T. (1994). *Legal, ethical and political issues in nursing*, Philadelphia: F. A. Davis.
2. Guido, G. W. (1997). *Legal issues in nursing* (2nd ed.). Stamford, Conn.: Appleton & Lange.
3. Beckmann, J. P. (1995). Problems associated with equipment and products. In *Nursing malpractice*. Seattle: University of Washington Press.
4. Bellaire General Hospital v. Campbell, 510 S.W.2d 94 (Tex. 1974).
5. Knowlton v. Deseret Medical, Inc., (1991).
6. Tammelleo, A. D. (1996). If equipment causes injury. *RN, 59*(1), 53.
7. Harris, A. V., and Ziel, S. E. (1996). Reporting requirements under the Safe Medical Devices Act. *AORN Journal, 64*(3), 460.
8. Dasse, P. S. (1991, December). Commentary: Improving the Safe Medical Devices Act. Online Forum. Available at bttp://www.rmf.org/w3961html.
9. American Association for Respiratory Care (1994). *Statement of ethics and professional conduct*. Available at http://www.aarc.org/professional resources/position statements/ethics htm. Dallas: American Association for Respiratory Care.
10. American Nurses Association (1985). *Code for nurses with interpretive statements*. Washington, D. C.: American Nurses Publishing.
11. American Physical Therapy Association (1991). *Code of ethics*. Available at http://www.apta.code of ethics.htm. Alexandria: American Physical Therapy Association.
12. Commission on Standards and Ethics (1994, July). *Occupational therapy code of ethics*. Bethesda: American Occupational Therapy Association.
13. Fiesta, J. (1997). Who's liable in equipment cases? *Nursing Management, 30*(4), 12–13, 15.

14. Gerlin, A. (1999, September 12). Widow's hunch reveals fatal hospital error. *The Times-Picayune Newspaper,* A-22.

15. Shinn, L. J. (Ed.) (1997). *Take control: A guide to risk management.* Chicago: Kirke-Van Orsdel, Inc.

16. Haddad, A. (1998). *Ethics in action. RN, 61*(9), 21.

17. Gaffney, T. (1997). Regulation of nursing practice. In L. J. Shinn (Ed.). *Take control: A guide to risk management.* Chicago: Kirke-Van Orsdel.

18. Quinn, C. (1998). Infusion devices: A bleeding vein of clinical negligence. *Journal of Nursing Management, 6*(4), 209–214.

19. Pearce v. Fetnstein, 754 E.Supp. 308, 309 (W.D.N.Y. 1990).

12

Patient Care Liability and Litigation

JOANN PIETRO, RN, JD

► **Key Chapter Concepts**

Patient Care
Nursing Home
Hospital
Rehabilitation Center
Psychiatric Center
Physical Therapy Center
Financial Reimbursement
Liability
Negligence

► **Objectives**

At the conclusion of this chapter, the reader should be able to:

1. Recognize potential areas of concern or liability areas.

2. Identify negligence and a negligent act.

3. Recognize how to avoid negligence.

4. Understand the litigation process.

INTRODUCTION

This chapter will explore the issues of patient care, liability, negligence, and litigation surrounding patient care.

PATIENT CARE

Patient contact is the most essential service that the allied health professional provides in the healthcare setting. The allied health professional has an obligation to practice safely and properly. At the current time, healthcare services are provided in multiple settings. The healthcare settings are as follows:

1. The **home** is where outpatient services for an acute or chronic medical condition are provided.
2. **Nursing homes** are the long-term care institutions that provide care for the chronically ill and elderly.
3. **Hospitals** are healthcare facilities where care is provided to patients who have emergency or urgent healthcare problems.
4. **Rehabilitation centers** are short-term care facilities where care is provided for the physically and mentally incapacitated.
5. **Psychiatric centers** are facilities for the care of the mentally ill.
6. **Physical therapy centers** or **clinics** are where outpatient recuperative services are provided.

DOCUMENTATION OF SERVICES

Financial Reimbursement

The financial reimbursement of institutions is directly associated with the services that are provided to the patients. The role of the allied health professional is to properly provide services that are ordered and to see that the services provided are documented.

▶ Case Scenario

A patient was admitted to Columbus Hospital by his attending physician for complaints of stomach pains. The treating physician knew that the patient had a history of alcohol abuse. The physician ordered that the patient be administered the medication Librium on an as needed basis for any signs of anxiety, which is the first sign of alcohol withdrawal. If alcohol withdrawal is not controlled, the patient could become delusional and cause harm to himself or others. The attending physician had the last actual contact with the patient at 5:00 p.m., at which time he left the patient in the hands of the nursing staff.

Although the patient initially did fairly well and was without complaint, his condition deteriorated over time. The night shift noticed that the patient was experiencing increasing anxiety. The nursing staff did not administer Librium as ordered or call the physician to notify him of the patient's change in condition. The nurses and nurses aides failed to closely monitor the patient.

The patient's anxiety continued. There were clear exhibitions of unusual or abnormal behavior by the patient. The patient verbally expressed anger at himself and others. He advised that he wished to leave the hospital to buy alcohol. He refused to comply with nursing instructions. He threatened the other patient in his room with an intravenous pole. The patient's behavior became so outrageous that a nurse's aide was placed outside the patient's room to keep a watchful eye on him. The patient's problem continued to escalate and ended when the patient jumped out of the window of his hospital room.

The patient fell several floors and landed on a roof extension below. Emergency services were provided. His life was saved, but he became a paraplegic. Before this incident, although he had an active drinking problem, he was a healthy, robust man without physical limitations or mental disability. Who was negligent? What were the negligent acts?

Documentation

Documentation of a service provided to the patient is as complex as writing a note in a patient's chart or as simple as preparing a bill for the services. Documentation of a service is dependent on which allied health professional provides the services. For instance, a nurse's aide records vital signs. A physical or respiratory therapist records in a patient's chart about a treatment. Other allied health professionals do not document in a patient's chart, but give information to a supervisor, nurse, or physician, who then enters information in the patient's chart. The requirements for documenting depend on the professional and the policies and procedures of the facility.

WHO ARE ALLIED HEALTH PROFESSIONALS

The allied healthcare professional plays a role in providing either direct or indirect services to patients (Boxes 12–1 and 12–2). Allied

---

BOX 12–1 • DIRECT SERVICES

1. Taking vital signs
2. Performing respiratory therapy
3. Performing physical therapy
4. Performing occupational therapy

BOX 12–2 • INDIRECT SERVICES

1. Assisting in a medical procedure
2. Assisting a nurse in providing a treatment to a patient
3. Handing instruments to a healthcare provider who is actually performing a procedure
4. Assisting a physical therapist in the transport of a patient

healthcare professionals who provide direct services or indirect services under the direction of a supervisor, registered nurse, dentist, or physician include the following:

1. Medical assistant
2. Respiratory therapist/respiratory technician
3. Rehabilitation/science professional—physical therapist, physical therapy assistant, occupational therapist, occupational assistant
4. Nursing assistants/nursing aides
5. Dental hygienist/dental technician
6. Radiologic technician/technologist
7. Ultrasound technician/technologist.

Examples of **direct** services include taking vital signs and performing respiratory therapy, physical therapy, or occupational therapy.

The allied healthcare professional might also provide **indirect** services. An example of indirect services includes assisting a physician or nurse during a treatment or medical procedure.

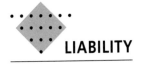

LIABILITY

Allied healthcare professionals are liable for their **negligent acts** which cause injuries to patients. Liability occurs in two ways:

1. Liability can arise from an act or omission by an allied healthcare professional.
2. Liability can arise when the allied healthcare professional participates or acts in a supervisory capacity in a negligent act committed by another healthcare provider.

The allied healthcare professional is negligent when he or she deviates from the accepted or **reasonable** allied health professional standard. For example, a physical therapist applies hot pack therapy treatment to a patient's extremity. The therapist must determine if the hot packs are of an even, consistent, and appropriate temperature to prevent patient burns. The act of applying a hot pack that burns the patient is considered negligent. The physical therapist has a duty to check the temperature prior to application, ensure patient safety, and prevent burns of extremities.

Faulty Equipment

If a nurse's aide or medical assistant is requested by a nurse to assist in the transport of a patient and is instructed to obtain a stretcher, the stretcher that is obtained should be in good working order. If the aide or assistant knows that the stretcher has a faulty wheel but utilizes it anyway, the aide or assistant may be held negligent if injury occurs. The law deems that the knowledge of faulty equipment puts the allied health professional on notice of the potential for possible injury to the patient. The aide or assistant has a duty to check equipment to see if it is in safe working order and to report faulty equipment.

Treatment Negligence

Another example of negligence involves a respiratory therapist or technician. For example, a therapist is assigned to administer a respiratory treatment to a fresh postoperative patient, Ms. Wong, who is on the telemetry unit. However, because the therapist fails to properly identify the patient, he does not realize that there are actually two patients on the telemetry unit with the last name of Wong. The patient that the therapist administers the treatment to has an untoward reaction which results in severe respiratory distress. The therapist is negligent for providing a treatment to the wrong patient. The therapist has a duty to properly identify a patient by checking the patient's full name, armband, or other means for patient identification. The therapist has also committed a battery by treating a patient for whom no order of treatment existed.

Standards of Care

To determine if the allied healthcare professional is conducting himself as a **reasonable** professional, the judge or jury determines if the professional practiced in accordance with the accepted standards in that particular specialty. Allied health professionals must conduct themselves in accordance with the applicable professional standards, rules, and regulations (see Box 12–3).

BOX 12–3 • SOURCES OF STANDARDS

The sources for standards of care include, but are not limited to, the following:

1. Allied healthcare professional associations

2. Rules and regulations set forth by the Joint Commission on Accreditation for Healthcare Organizations (JCAHO)

3. Policies, procedures, bylaws, rules, and regulations set forth by an institution or employer

4. Current medical literature and authoritative textbooks

5. Experts in the field

6. Job descriptions

7. Instruction manuals

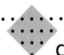

COMMON AREAS OF NEGLIGENCE

The allied health professional can breach the standards of care in numerous ways. Examples of the primary area of concern for some of the allied healthcare professional groups are listed in Boxes 12–4 through 12–7.

Nursing and medical assistants share the same areas of potential negligence. They can avoid negligence by conducting themselves **reasonably** when providing patient services. The nursing or medical assistant must be careful when assisting patients. They should always give adequate physical support and ensure that pathways are clear. The nursing or medical assistant who is responsible for bedridden patients must turn patients frequently and safely and comfortably position the patient to avoid decubitus ulcers (bedsores). Also, when positioning a patient on an examining room table or in a bed, the assistant must protect the patient from injury.

When using equipment, the nursing and medical assistant must check the equipment to see that it is in good working order. The assistant is not required to act as an engineer. Rather this means that the assistant must use common sense when securing or utilizing

BOX 12–4 • COMMON AREAS OF NEGLIGENCE FOR NURSING ASSISTANTS

1. Failure to properly assist a patient while ambulating, getting out of bed or during transport
2. Failure to properly position a patient
3. Unsafe placement or positioning of equipment or medical devices
4. Failure to properly monitor a patient under observation
5. Failure to report changes in a patient's condition to a nurse or physician or other appropriate healthcare provider
6. Failure to adhere to facility rules, regulations, policies or procedures
7. Failure to properly perform a task such as assisting a patient with feeding or bathing or providing other patient contact
8. Failure to properly provide equipment to a physician or nurse who the aid is assisting
9. Failure to chart, report or record information accurately, promptly, and properly
10. Failure to recognize equipment failure or problems resulting in patient injury

BOX 12–5 • COMMON AREAS OF NEGLIGENCE FOR MEDICAL ASSISTANTS

1. Failure to properly assist a patient while ambulating, getting out of bed or during transport
2. Failure to properly and safely position a patient
3. Unsafe placement or positioning of equipment or medical devices
4. Failure to monitor a patient during required observation
5. Failure to adhere to the employer's rules, policies, regulations, and procedures
6. Negligently providing equipment to a healthcare provider during a procedure
7. Failure to give proper advice or instructions to a patient
8. Failure to refer inquiry directly to the registered nurse, physician or other appropriate healthcare provider

BOX 12–6 • COMMON AREAS OF NEGLIGENCE FOR RESPIRATORY THERAPISTS/RESPIRATORY TECHNICIANS

1. Failure to timely and properly perform a treatment
2. Participating in a treatment which is negligently provided by another healthcare provider
3. Failure to properly check the working order of all equipment which is utilized
4. The use of faulty equipment
5. Failure to adhere to a facility's policies, procedures, practices, and protocols
6. Failure to recognize and/or report a change in respiratory status to a supervisor or physician
7. Improper or inadequate documentation

BOX 12–7 • COMMON AREAS OF NEGLIGENCE FOR PHYSICAL THERAPISTS, OCCUPATIONAL THERAPISTS, AND ASSISTANTS

1. Failure to timely and properly perform a treatment
2. Participating in a treatment which is negligently provided by another healthcare provider
3. Failure to properly check the working order of all equipment which is going to be utilized
4. The use of faulty equipment
5. Failure to adhere to a hospital's policies, procedures, practices, and protocols
6. Failure to recognize and/or report a change in status to a supervisor or the physician
7. Improper or inadequate charting

equipment. Equipment that has been previously known to malfunction or has an obviously broken part should not be utilized. If placing equipment in a patient's room, it should be done properly and safely. Extension cords, furniture, or rugs should be not be left in the patient's walkway or in areas that can cause injury.

The assistant assigned to monitor the patient must do so diligently. If the patient is to be observed at set intervals, then this must be done and documented. If restraints are to be regularly checked, then the assistant needs to physically accomplish this monitoring by touching and properly observing and documenting. If a change in the patient's condition is noticed, this must also be reported to a supervisor.

Tasks should be delivered in accordance with the employer's protocols. The employer has written policies to insure the quality of services. Policies are used to give direction to employees. If assisting a patient in eating, hot beverages must not be left in unsafe positions so that they can spill on the patient.

The assistant must accurately record or provide information to a supervisor regarding a patient. If there is an obligation to chart information, then it must be done in a timely fashion so that other healthcare providers have the information available to them. Assistants should not give nursing or medical instructions or advise patients. Any questions from the patient should be communicated to the nurse, physician, or other appropriate healthcare provider.

LIABILITY AND LITIGATION

If the allied healthcare professional acts negligently, there is a significant chance of being sued. Patients have grown to be a litigious group. Some are quick to sue for actual wrongdoing or perceived wrongdoing. There is a high but unrealistic expectation on the part of patients that all of the contact they have with the healthcare system will be positive and beneficial to them. A negative experience, even one that results in minor injury, is enough for some patients to file a lawsuit or a complaint with professional boards.

Financial compensation is a patient's redress for injuries that have been sustained. Patients can receive compensation for actual physical injuries, medical expenses, lost wages, pain and suffering, emotional distress, mental anguish, and loss of consortium, just to name a few. If sued, you will be served with a copy of the lawsuit or a letter outlining plaintiffs, defendants, and allegations of breaches of the standard of care. Some states have a different pre-trial process whereby the plaintiff must present the case to a medical review panel for review prior to actually filing the claim with the courts. The claim must be given immediately to the employer. In turn, the employer gives the paperwork to the insurance carrier. The insurance carrier then assigns an attorney to the healthcare provider. It is not unusual for the allied healthcare professional to be represented by the same attorney that represents the employer, the hospital, nursing home, doctor's office or clinic. If you have your own professional liability policy, contact your insurance carrier.

The attorney who is assigned to you will represent your interest. Once you are sued, you should not discuss the case with anyone except your attorney. All costs associated with the lawsuit are paid by the insurance company. Costs associated with the lawsuit include attorneys' fees, litigation costs (such as costs for experts, documents, and exhibits), court costs, and trial costs. More importantly, the insurance pays for any settlement of the case. It also pays a judgment if the case goes to trial and a jury awards the patient money.

To avoid being sued, the allied health professional must practice defensively. You must be vigilant and conduct yourself as a **"reasonable"** allied healthcare professional. If you are unsure or do not know the policy, practices, or protocol for a specific treatment or procedure, then you must seek help from someone who is more knowledgeable.

The healthcare environment can be a dangerous environment. Many allied health professionals work in areas of health care where there is a shortage of help. Others work in critical or emergency settings which have inherent liability because of the ever present fast pace at which services are delivered. Everyone must respond reasonably even during times which are truly life or death situations. Allied healthcare professionals may also be in settings where their coworkers are not adequately trained.

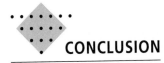

CONCLUSION

In conclusion, the allied healthcare professional must know and identify areas of potential liability. The case scenario in this chapter indicates an area of potential liability for the nursing assistant. The nursing assistant who was instructed by the nurses to monitor and observe the patient failed to adequately do so. The patient jumped out of the window of his hospital room with the nurse's aide sitting immediately outside of his hospital room door. The nurse's aide failed to observe a marked increase of anxiety and expression of communication by the patient of his intent to cause harm to himself. The nurse's aide failed to properly observe the patient by not watching him more closely and allowing him to exit through the hospital room window, falling and resulting in severe and permanent injury. The nurse's aide should have performed checks more frequently or should have observed the patient at his bedside. The aide should have been instructed to actually stay in the patient's room and should have promptly reported any change in the patient's condition to the supervisor.

PERTINENT POINTS

1. Being able to recognize a potential wrongdoing or negligent act and knowing the areas of potential legal exposure can decrease your involvement.

2. Patient care issues and medical equipment problems are two areas of potential litigation.

3. Communication between the professionals, patient, and family is an important key to decreasing potential litigation.

STUDY QUESTIONS

1. What are three areas of practice commonly breached by nursing assistants?

2. List five sources for standards of care for allied health professionals.

3. How can medical assistants decrease potential liability in their practice? Describe five ways.

4. What are things that can be done to decrease liability when using medical equipment?

5. What are five areas of potential legal exposure for the respiratory therapist technician?

6. Describe areas of negligence that you have found in a case obtained from the law library or the internet in the area of physical therapy.

7. List and describe six common healthcare settings.

8. Describe common areas of negligence where nursing assistants may be held accountable.

9. What are concerns for dental hygienists and technicians when dealing with patients?

10. How can radiological technologists and technicians decrease exposure to litigation?

13

The Basics of Alternative Dispute Resolution

TONIA DANDRY AIKEN, RN, BSN, JD
PAULA DIMEO GRANT, RN, BSN, MA, JD
DIANE TRACE WARLICK, RN, BSN, JD
AND JAMES B. AIKEN, MD, MHA, FACEP

▶ **Key Chapter Concepts**

Alternative Dispute Resolution
Mediation
Arbitration
Dispute
Negotiation
Communication
Open-Ended Questions
Closed-Ended Questions
Nonverbal Communication

▶ **Objectives**

At the conclusion of this chapter, the reader should be able to:

1. Discuss the reasons to use alternative dispute resolution (ADR).

2. Define mediation and arbitration.

3. Discuss the communication process and its role in ADR.

4. Define negotiation.

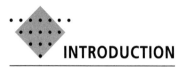

INTRODUCTION

Disputes take the form of arguments, challenges, contests, lawsuits, fights, or even war. The alternative dispute resolution (ADR) movement is the process that focuses on alternative ways to resolve disputes among parties, including employers and employees or others in confrontational situations. Disputes occur constantly and are resolved daily, some in a more effective manner than others. The ability to resolve these disputes at an early stage avoids the following:

1. **Lengthy court delays;**
2. **Uncontrollable costs;**
3. **Unwanted publicity;**
4. **Ill will; and**
5. **Win-lose courtroom confrontation.**

In addition, quick resolution protects ongoing relationships by using impartial, neutral third parties to resolve the dispute. The ADR movement resolves conflict through the following:

1. Negotiation
2. Mediation
3. Arbitration
4. Communication.

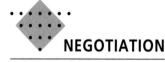

NEGOTIATION

Negotiation is any communication used in an attempt to achieve a goal, approval, or action by another. Those in allied health use negotiation skills in numerous situations with patients, families, coworkers, and employers.

We begin the act of negotiation at a very young age. When you were young and asked your parents for four cookies and they said one and you finally settled for two, you were negotiating. Negotiating takes place every time two or more individuals work out an argument of any kind. It may be formal or informal.

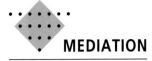

MEDIATION

Both the private and public sectors are using mediation to resolve disputes. For example, government agencies have been charged with investigating and adjudicating workplace claims. The U.S. Equal Employment Opportunity Commission, the U.S. Postal Service, and state agencies are experimenting with the use of mediation programs as a means to end disputes. The United States Supreme Court recently held that employment contracts may require arbitration of employer-employee disputes [1].

Mediation can be similarly compelled by contract. **Mediation is the process in which a neutral third party (who may be an attorney, judge, or other person trained in mediation techniques) facilitates and assists the parties in resolving a dispute** (see Box 13–1). The fundamental principal of mediation is self-determination. Mediation relies on the ability of the parties to reach a voluntary uncoerced agreement. The mediator may offer a possible resolution for discus-

---

BOX 13–1 • MEDIATION

The mediation process allows disputants the opportunity to:

1. Address past conflicts and problems
2. Address future relationships
3. Discuss in detail the problems in a nonthreatening environment
4. Make informed, voluntary, and uncoerced decisions
5. Have access to the process no matter what their level of economic status is in the community
6. Discuss the conflicts with expectations of confidentiality
7. Have access to legal counsel
8. Empower the parties to resolve disputes, since they are the decision-makers

sion, help the parties explore the options, and identify issues and provide information. There is more than one model for mediation, but most recognize at least the following stages to the process:

1. **Introduction to the process, parties, and general rules**
2. **Information gathering**
3. **Identification of parties' interests**
4. **Brainstorming—generating ideas and options**
5. **Negotiation and selection of appropriate resolution**
6. **Clarification and finalization of the agreement.**

This process is commonly used to resolve medical malpractice claims, personal injury claims, and employee disputes. It is the least adversarial, assists the parties in identifying the real issues, and offers options for settlement. The parties maintain control of the outcome.

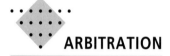

ARBITRATION

Arbitration is the process of resolving issues in conflict in a more structured setting like formal litigation. There can be one arbitrator or a panel of arbitrators, who can award damages, interest, attorney's fees, and punitive damages (if allowed by law). Also, in this process discovery is allowed and witness lists are produced. Informal rules of evidence are used. Arbitration is usually voluntary but can be mandated by law for specific disputes, such as those involving labor and unions. The arbitrator, who is a neutral party, should provide a written opinion and award that includes the type of dispute and issues decided. Remedies should be consistent with statutes or the law that would apply if the case were tried in court.

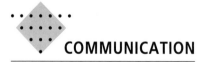

COMMUNICATION

If you are in a situation in which the patient has told you that he wants to live and requests that you help him in every way possible, but he then refuses to get out of bed or take his medication, what message is he really communicating through his actions?

BOX 13–2 • SAMPLE QUESTION TYPES

Open-Ended Questions

1. How do you feel today?
2. How are you dealing with the death of your sister?

Closed-Ended Questions

1. Did you eat your breakfast?
2. Does your right foot hurt this morning?

Communication is the process by which a person conveys his needs, wants, feelings, or ideas through verbal or nonverbal means. **Listening** is a key to effective communication. **Open-ended** and **closed-ended questions** (see Box 13–2) elicit information that can be useful in the communication process and ADR.

In addition to verbal communication, the healthcare provider must be attentive to **nonverbal communication**. Nonverbal communication can take the form of the following:

1. **Body language with your eyes, face, hands, legs, arms, and posture;**
2. **Clothing; and**
3. **Hygiene.**

Your body language also reveals many feelings: for example, rolling your eyes (as if in disbelief), tapping your fingers (anxiety), or crossing your arms (a defensive position).

Professionals also dress in a certain manner: sloppy clothing and poor hygiene (uncombed hair or unshaven) present a certain image or picture to the outside world.

In ADR, the mediator or arbitrator is trained to detect body language and communication signals that can stall or cause the process to fail. It is his or her job to facilitate the process and continue to achieve progress in the negotiations and, hopefully, to conclude the matter.

Both communication and negotiation skills must be learned by the healthcare provider and are used in the process of alternative dispute resolution. ADR is a solution to timely and efficiently conclude complicated, costly, and time-consuming conflicts in the healthcare arena.

PERTINENT POINTS

1. Alternative dispute resolution provides alternative ways to resolve disputes in the form of mediation and arbitration.
2. Communication skills are needed to effectively negotiate.
3. Negotiation is used in numerous situations with patients, family, coworkers, and employer-employee situations.

STUDY QUESTIONS

1. Look at a television show and identify five types of communication—verbal or nonverbal—used by the characters.
2. Develop a scenario that involves a dispute between

    a. Coworkers

    b. Employer-employee

    c. Patient and provider

    d. Insurance company and staff.

    Decide and discuss how you approach resolution of the disputes.
3. Have a local mediator talk to your class about techniques used.
4. Discuss body language and five types of signals that a person conveys through body language.

REFERENCE

1. *Circuit City, Inc. v. Adams*, No. 99-1379 (March 21, 2001).

RESOURCES

1. Alessandra, T. & Hunsacker, P. (1993). *Communicating at Work*. New York: Simon and Schuster.
2. Dauer, E. et al. (2000). *Health care dispute resolution manual—Techniques for avoiding litigation*. Gaithersburg: Aspen Publishers.
3. Donaldson, M. & Donaldson, M. (1996). *Negotiating for dummies*. Chicago: IDG Books Worldwide, Inc.
4. Kovach, K. (1994). *Mediation-principles and practice*. St. Paul: West Group.
5. Model Standards of Practice for Mediators. ABA, SPIDR and AAA.

ADDITIONAL INFORMATION

1. American Arbitration Association, 335 Madison Avenue, Floor 10, New York, NY 10017-4605 (212-716-5800; 800-778-7879; 212-716-5905).

2. American Bar Association, www.abanet.org. Section of Dispute Resolution, 740 Fifteenth Street, Washington, DC 20005 (202-662-1680; 202-662-1683 (Fax); email: dispute@abanet.org).

3. Society of Professionals in Dispute Resolution (SPIDR), 1527 New Hampshire Ave., N.W., Third Floor, Washington, DC 20036 (202-667-9700; 202-265-1968 (Fax); e-mail: spiddr@spidr.org).

4. The American Association of Nurse Attorneys, 7794 Grow Drive, Pensacola, FL 32514 (850-484-8762; 1-800-538-2262; email: taana@puetzame.com).

Glossary

Administrative Law: Codifies the interactions between the citizens and the agencies, provides for certain police power to the agencies to enforce the regulations, and governs the agencies themselves.

Administrative Remedies: Monetary fines, required education, loss of license to practice or restrictions in practice.

Agencies: Enact rules and regulations that become administrative law.

Aggregate Amount: The total amount that the insurer pays during the policy period, usually 1 year, regardless of the number of incidents, claims, claimants or defendants.

Alternative Dispute Resolution (ADR): The process that focuses on alternative ways to resolve disputes among parties, including employers and employees or others in confrontational situations.

Against Medical Advice (AMA): Refers to situations where the patient wishes to leave the facility.

Arbitrary: Subject to individual will or judgment without restriction; capricious.

Arbitration: The process of resolving issues in conflict in a more structured setting like formal litigation.

Assault: Placing someone in immediate fear or apprehension of a harmful or noxious touching without that person's consent. (Intentional tort)

Autonomy: Independence or freedom as of the will or one's actions.

Battery: A harmful or offensive touching of another without his or her consent or without a legally justifiable reason. (Intentional tort)

Beneficence: Doing good or kindness. In bioethical terms, the principle of beneficence means that we as healthcare professionals should always try to help patients and make their situation better.

Bioethics: Ethics that deal with patients and health care.

Bioethical Principles: (1) Patient's autonomy; (2) beneficence; (3) nonmaleficence; (4) justice; and (5) professional ethics.

Breach of Confidentiality: Occurs when someone who has legitimate access to health information about a patient shares it with others who have no legitimate reason to know.

Checks and Balances: Limits imposed on all branches of a government by vesting in each branch the right to amend or veto each other.

Civil Code: Developed from Roman law codified by the legislature.

Civil Law: Case is brought by an individual or entity against another for harm based in tort, contract, labor or privacy.

Claims-Made Policy: A type of professional liability insurance policy that covers injuries only if the injury occurs in the policy period and the claim is reported to the insurance company during the policy period or during the "tail."

Claims-Made Trigger: Coverage is provided for any claim made while the policy is in force.

Clinical Laboratory Improvement Amendment (CLIA): Sets forth extensive conditions or standards that laboratories must meet to be certified by the United States Department of Health and Human Services.

Common Knowledge Exception: The defendant's negligence is so grossly apparent or the treatment is so common that a lay person can readily appraise it using his everyday knowledge.

Common Law: Developed on a case by case basis from England when the king decided in his "divine right."

Communication: The process by which a person conveys his needs, wants, feelings, or ideas through verbal or nonverbal means.

Competence: The ability to provide a level of care according to a standard of care and according to the profession's code of ethics.

Competency: The ability to understand the nature and consequences of the medical procedure.

CPC: (1) Computerize patient record or (2) confidential personal code.

Consent: To permit, approve or comply.

Contribution: When there are others who, although not named in a claim, bear at least some responsibility for the incident.

Criminal Law: A case is brought by the state or federal government for violation of written criminal code or statute.

Declarations Page: Frequently called the *"dec"* page in insurance jargon, this is where the policy lists the name(s) of the person or institution insured.

Defamation: False communication to a third party that damages that person's reputation. Libel (written) and slander (oral) communications, (Quasi-intentional tort) are two forms of defamation.

Defendant: The person or entity sued.

Dental Hygienist: A licensed primary healthcare professional, oral health educator and clinician who, as a co-therapist, provides preventative, educational, and therapeutic services supporting total health for the control of oral diseases and the promotion of oral health.

Direct Services: Taking vital signs, performing respiratory therapy, physical therapy or occupational therapy.

Discriminatory: Showing prejudice or partiality.

Disciplinary Action: Action taken against a professional's license. Usually brought because the professional has caused an unsafe condition or environment for the patient.

Electronic Charting: Computerized documentation.

Endorsements: Added provisions that delete or modify the coverage provided in the standard provisions or "policy jacket" part of the policy. These provisions, sometimes called *"riders,"* address items that apply to the insured's specific situation.

Ethics: Declarations of what is right or wrong and of what ought to be.

Ethics Committee: Committee created to deal with ethical problems and dilemmas in patient care.

Excess Coverage: The amount the insurer is obligated to pay after the second policy has paid.

Exclusions: All of the circumstances for which coverage is not provided.

Executive Branch: President of the United States or Governor of an individual state. Can propose laws, veto laws proposed by the legislature, enforce the laws, and establish agencies.

Expert: A person with knowledge, experience, and expertise in a field of practice used in litigation to support or defend litigant's position.

Expert Testimony: Generally required to establish the applicable standard of care in malpractice actions.

False Imprisonment: The unlawful detention of a person through chemical, physical or emotional means. (Intentional tort)

Felonies: More serious crimes punishable by relatively large fines and/or imprisonment for more than 1 year and, in some states, death.

Flow Sheet: A table that consists of information in columns; a graphic sheet designed so that several days' worth of patient data are on one form.

Focus Charting: Uses a format of having a column for the focus or problem. The note is then organized into D for data, A for action, and R for response.

Fourteenth Amendment: Mandates that no state shall deprive a person of life, liberty or property without due process of law.

Good Samaritan Law: Protects those that provide health care for an emergency or disaster without reimbursement.

Graphic Sheet: A document designed so that several days worth of data are on one form, e.g., vital sign sheet listing temperature, pulse, and respirations.

Hospitals: Healthcare facilities where care is provided to patients who have emergency or urgent healthcare problems.

Incident Report: Also known as Variance or Occurrence Report. Documentation of incidents that contain an objective factual description of events.

Incompetence: The failing of moral commitment in upholding the code of ethics.

Indemnification: The insured contends that some other person was totally responsible for an incident and, therefore, that other person should reimburse or indemnify the insured for the entire amount paid to claimant(s).

Independent Contractor: A person who is self-employed and who enters into contracts to provide professional services to various entities such as hospitals, doctors' offices, and/or individual clients.

Indirect Services: Assisting a physician or nurse during a treatment or medical procedure.

Informed Consent: The process of providing adequate information for a patient in an understandable fashion to enable the patient to make a knowledgeable decision about whether to accept or refuse a proposed treatment. Disclosure requirements include: (1) type of procedure to be performed; (2) nature and purpose of proposed treatment; (3) material risks and consequences; (4) alternatives; and (5) consequences of no treatment.

In Personam Jurisdiction: A term which means that the court has jurisdiction over the person.

In Rem Jurisdiction: A term which means that the court has jurisdiction over the property or thing itself rather than over the people involved.

Insurance: A contract between the insured and the insurer that protects the insured from a specified loss.

Insuring Agreement of Insuring Clause: States the agreement between the insurer and the insured as to what coverage is provided. The clause briefly states what type of claim, (e.g., damages due to injury) the insurer is obligated to pay and under what conditions, (e.g., injury due to acts or omissions of the insured) while the policy is in force.

Intake and Output Sheets: Documentation sheets for the healthcare provider to record the intake for intravenous fluid solutions, hyperalimentation, etc., and output, e.g., urine, feces, gastric contents, etc.

Intentional Infliction of Emotional Distress: In order to establish the tort of intentional infliction of emotional distress, the plaintiff must establish that the defendant's conduct is outrageous and beyond the bounds of common decency. Insulting behavior is not enough. The actions must be egregious.

Intentional Torts: Require that there be an intentional interference with one's person, reputation, or property (e.g., assault, battery, false imprisonment).

Interrogatories: Written questions that must be answered under oath.

Invasion of Privacy: The tort of unjustifiably intruding upon another's right of privacy by appropriating his or her name or likeness, unreasonably interfering with his or her seclusion, publishing private facts, or publicly placing a person in a false light. (Quasi-intentional tort)

JCAHO: Joint Commission on Accreditation of Healthcare Organizations.

Judicial Branch: Court system. Interprets legislation and may overrule laws and actions of the executive branch.

Judicial System: The court system (including federal courts and state courts) which develops and interprets statutory law.

Justice: Treating everyone fairly.

Kardex: An abbreviated listing of the care elements specific to the patient. The kardex commonly defines the type of diet, the patient's activity level, the amount of assistance the patient needs for bathing, and the treatments that are to be performed.

Law: The foundation of statutes, rules, and regulations that govern people, relationships, behaviors, and interactions with the state, society, and federal government.

Legislative Branch: The House of Representatives and Senate of the United States and any similar legislature of a state that develops statutory law.

Liability: An individual's responsibility of his conduct for failure to meet a standard of care or for failure to perform a duty that causes harm to a client.

Liability Insurance: Insurance that protects personal and professional assets in the event of professional liability and malpractice suit.

Libel: Written defamatory statements.

Living Will: A document, which may be handwritten, in which the patient describes his/her wishes regarding life-sustaining treatment. The document only takes effect if (1) it complies with the requirements of the law of the state in which the patient is located and (2) the patient is incompetent to make healthcare decisions.

Malpractice: Dereliction of professional duty through negligence, ignorance or criminal intent.

Mediation: The process in which a neutral third party (who may be an attorney, judge, or other person trained in mediation techniques) facilitates and assists the parties in resolving a dispute.

Medical Device: A broad term encompassing such items as implants, single use of disposable devices, instruments, machines, apparatus, and reagents.

Minor: An individual under the age of 18.

Misdemeanors: Lesser crimes with fines established by the state, which are usually modest, and/or imprisonment of less than 1 year.

Moral Dilemma: Occurs when moral ideas conflict.

Morals: Ideas about right and wrong.

Negligence: The failure to use such care as a reasonably prudent and careful person would use under similar circumstances; it is the doing of some act which a person of ordinary prudence would not have done under similar circumstances or failure to do what a person of ordinary prudence would have done under similar circumstances. **Elements of Negligence:** (1) Duty; (2) breach of duty; (3) proximate cause; and (4) harm or damage.

Negotiation: Any communication used in an attempt to achieve a goal, approval or action by another.

Nonmaleficence: Do no harm. In bioethical terms, the principle of nonmaleficence means that healthcare professionals should avoid harming a patient.

Nursing Home: A long-term care institution that provides care for the chronically ill and elderly.

Occurrence Policy: Professional liability insurance policy that covers injuries that occur during the period covered by the policy even though they may be reported outside the policy period.

Ordinary Negligence: Conduct which involves undue risk of harm to others.

OSHA: Occupational Safety and Health Administration.

Physical Therapy Centers: Where outpatient recuperative services are provided.

PIE Charting: Structures the progress note into P for problem, I for intervention, and E for evaluation.

Plaintiff: The person or entity bringing the suit or claim.

Plan of Care: May be recorded in a hospital or nursing home in the form of a nursing care plan. The care plan usually defines the patient's problems, the outcomes or goals that are to be achieved, and the interventions or steps to be carried out to achieve the outcomes.

Policy Provisions: Sometimes called the "policy jacket," this section sets forth the generic provisions that are found in most policies of the same type.

Precedent: A legal decision serving as an authoritative rule in similar cases that follow.

Premium: Money contributed by each insured member and pooled by the insurer into a fund.

Prior Acts: Incidents that occurred prior to the beginning effective date of the policy.

Private Institutions: Are not supported by state revenues and typically receive financial support from private funding.

Product Liability: Different from malpractice in that the patient may not have to prove a deviation from a standard of care if the courts apply a **strict liability standard.** With a strict liability standard, the equipment's manufacturer may be held liable.

Professional Negligence: A negligent act or omission by a healthcare provider in the rendering of professional services, which is the proximate cause of a personal injury or wrongful death, provided that the services are within the scope of services for which the provider is licensed and which are not within any restriction imposed by the licensing agency or licensed hospital.

Psychiatric Centers: Institutions for the mentally ill.

Public Academic Institutions: Are affiliated with state government, are deemed state institutions, and are supported by state revenues.

Radiology Technologists: Usually employed in hospitals and cancer centers to deliver radiation to patients for therapeutic purposes.

Rehabilitation Centers: Short-term care facilities where care is provided for the physically and mentally incapacitated.

Res Ipsa Loquitur: Legal doctrine that means, "The thing speaks for itself." Often used in operating room malpractice cases where sponges, needles or hemostats are left in the patient.

Respondeat Superior: Legal doctrine that means, "Let the master answer." Used to hold the employer responsible and liable for the negligent acts of its employees.

Safe Medical Device Act of 1990 (SMDA): A **medical device** is a broad term encompassing such items as implants, single use of disposable devices, instruments, machines, apparatus, and reagents. The **Safe Medical Device Act** provides rules and regulations for the safety and reporting of medical devices.

Self-insurance: Some healthcare institutions elect to **self-insure** in accordance with state laws. The employer provides evidence that it has sufficient funds set aside to satisfy a successful claim.

Slander: Spoken defamatory statements.

SOAP Format: This system consists of a problem list and progress notes. The problem list is an ongoing listing of the patient's current and resolved problems. The progress note is broken down into four components: S (subjective), O (objective), A (assessment), and P (plan).

Sovereign Immunity: Is a defense that protects a federal or state employee when acting within the scope of employment.

Spoilation: The intentional destruction of evidence which, when established, allows the court to instruct the jury that it may infer that the lost or damaged evidence was unfavorable to the party responsible for the spoilation.

Standard of Care: A measure of the care that a reasonable and sensible person would use in the same situation.

Stare Decisis: "To stand by things decided" or to adhere to the decided case.

Statement of the Agreement: This is often called the *"insuring agreement"* or *"insuring clause"* and states the agreement between the insurer and the insured as to what coverage is provided.

Statute of Limitations: Used as a defense to a tort action. The statute requires that a claim be filed within a specific amount of time.

Statutory Law: Laws that are codified and impact all citizens of the state.

Subpoena Duces Tecum: A document attorneys direct to a custodian commanding the custodian to appear for a deposition and produce a patient's treatment record or other pertinent documents. State and federal courts have specific rules addressing the proper form, appropriate service, and other requirements necessary for the subpoena to be valid.

Surrogate Decision-Maker: A person permitted under state law to consent to medical treatment on a patient's behalf when the patient is incapable of doing so.

Tail Coverage Policy: An uninterrupted extension of the insurance policy period, also known as the extended reporting endorsement.

Tort: A civil wrong, other than breach of contract. The word tort is derived from an old Norman word meaning "wrong." A tort is a harm against a person, whereas a crime is a harm against the state.

Trespass to Land: Occurs when a person, without the consent of the owner, enters onto another's land or causes anyone or anything to enter the land or premises.

Umbrella Coverage: Is purchased in addition to a basic liability policy. It provides additional limit amounts and/or adds coverage for events not covered in the basic policy.

Vicarious Liability: Wherein the acts or omissions of the employee are imputed to the employer, so that the employer can be found liable for them.

X-Ray Technician: Only uses ionizing radiation for diagnostic purposes and has specific training to perform x-rays of the chest, extremities, gastrointestinal (GI), genitourinary (GU), leg-podiatric, skull, or torso-skeletal categories.

Index

Note: Page numbers followed by the letter b refer to boxed material.